MOVE

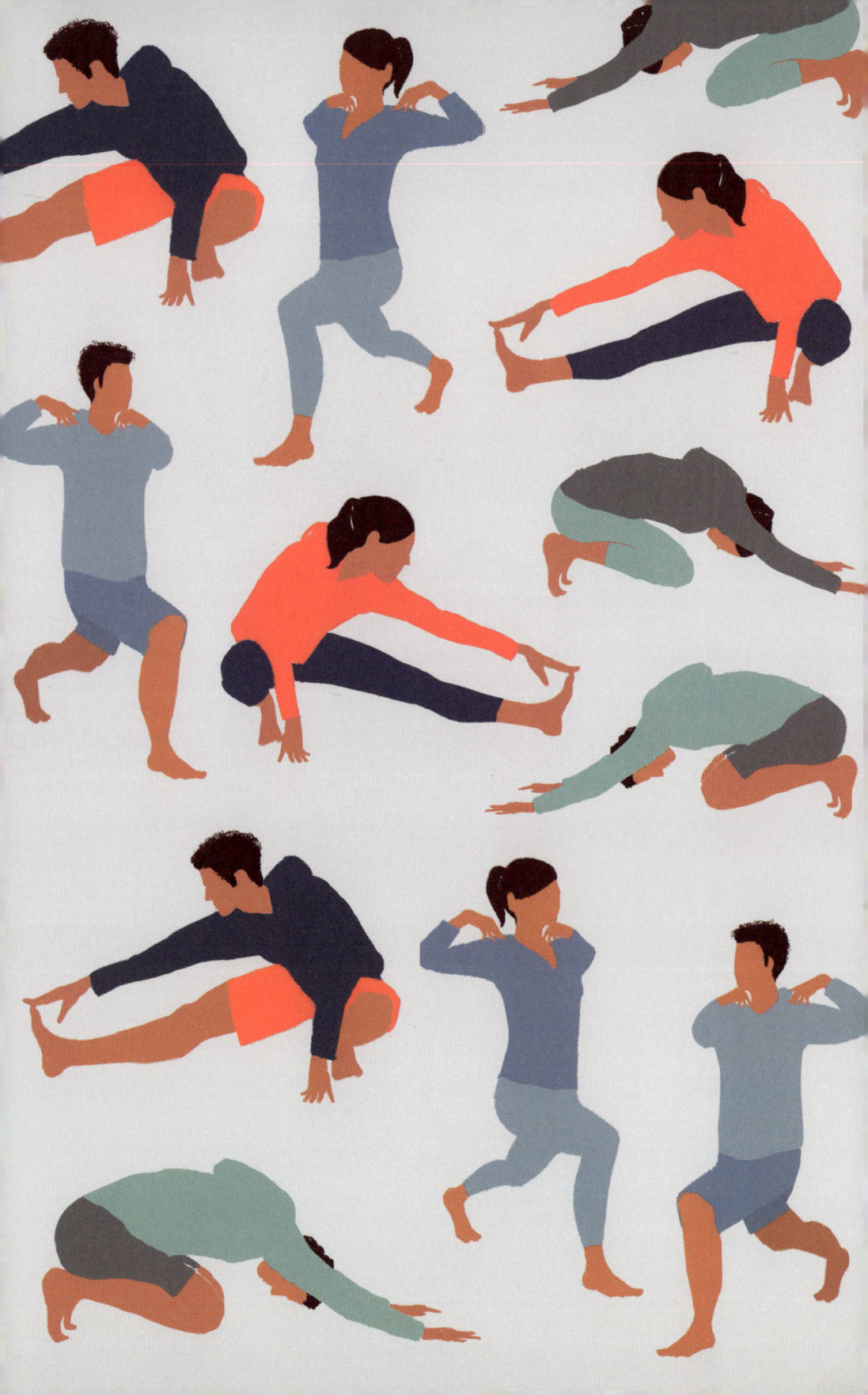

MOVE

Free Your Body Through Stretching Movement

Lexie Williamson

BLOOMSBURY SPORT
LONDON · OXFORD · NEW YORK · NEW DELHI · SYDNEY

BLOOMSBURY SPORT
Bloomsbury Publishing Plc
50 Bedford Square, London, WC1B 3DP, UK

BLOOMSBURY, BLOOMSBURY SPORT and the Diana logo are trademarks
of Bloomsbury Publishing Plc

First published in Great Britain 2020

Copyright © Lexie Williamson, 2020
Photography by Henry Hunt, 2020
Illustrations © Anna Morrison

Lexie Williamson has asserted her right under the Copyright, Designs and Patents Act, 1988,
to be identified as Author of this work.

For legal purposes the Acknowledgements on page 175 constitute an extension
of this copyright page.

All rights reserved. No part of this publication may be reproduced or transmitted in any form or by
any means, electronic or mechanical, including photocopying, recording, or any information storage or
retrieval system, without prior permission in writing from the publishers.

No responsibility for loss caused to any individual or organization acting on or refraining from action
as a result of the material in this publication can be accepted by Bloomsbury or the author.

Bloomsbury Publishing Plc does not have any control over, or responsibility for, any third-party web-
sites referred to or in this book. All internet addresses given in this book were correct at the time of
going to press. The author and publisher regret any inconvenience caused if addresses have changed
or sites have ceased to exist, but can accept no responsibility for any such changes.

A catalogue record for this book is available from the British Library
Library of Congress Cataloguing-in-Publication data has been applied for.

ISBN: TPB: 978-1-4729-7489-1; eBook: 978-1-4729-7490-7

2 4 6 8 10 9 7 5 3 1

Typeset in Gill Sans by Lee-May Lim
Printed and bound in China by Toppan Leefung Printing

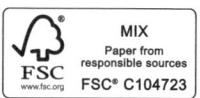

To find out more about our authors and books visit www.bloomsbury.com
and sign up for our newsletters.

CONTENTS

INTRODUCTION   06

THE MOVES   30
- 1: Back Mobility   34
- 2: Cat Play   41
- 3: Unstick the Hips   48
- 4: Lunge Flow   55
- 5: Hamstring Releasing   62
- 6: Shoulder Flossing   69

GENTLE MOVES   76

ADVANCED MOVES   122

MOVING FORWARD   168
OUR MOVERS   170
ACKNOWLEDGEMENTS   175
ABOUT THE AUTHOR   176

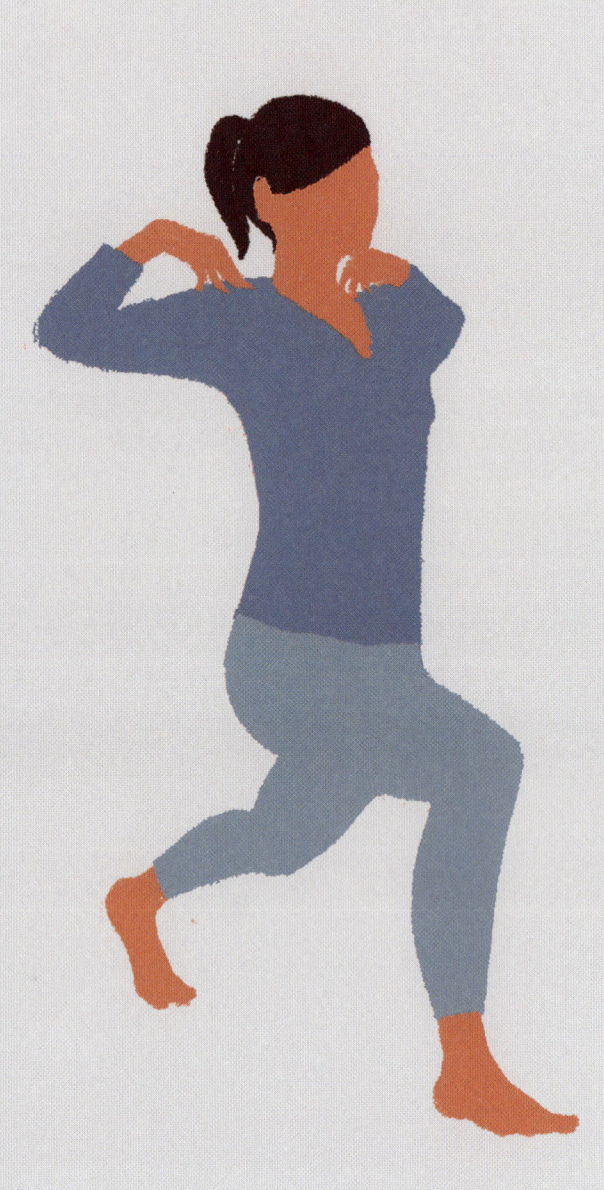

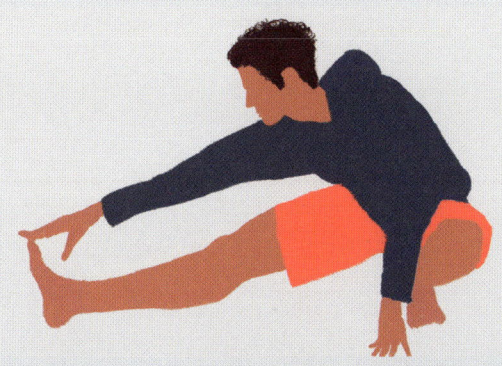

INTRODUCTION

Welcome to *Move*, a complete system of 'freeing up' the body through movement for anyone wanting to be less stiff or stuck, and more supple. These techniques will help you to regain precious long-lost flexibility, but also to stand tall, move better and (most importantly) to *feel* better.

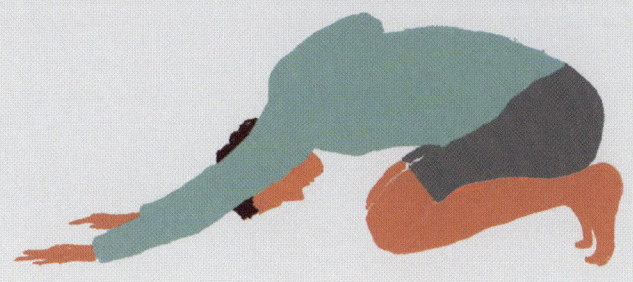

INTRODUCTION

Our bodies are designed to move – and move a lot – through all planes of motion, such as forward bending, twisting and side bending. As children, we relished this freedom as we tumbled, ran, flipped and cartwheeled without limits. Yet as adults, our jobs, responsibilities and lifestyles rarely allow us to enjoy the kind of multidirectional movement we once did without thinking.

Maybe you sit for eight hours a day hunched over a laptop. Perhaps you are frequently behind the wheel as the family taxi driver, or are studying for important exams. This enforced stillness is often an unavoidable element of our busy modern lives, but can lead to a gradual restriction of movement and muscular tension – thanks to the 'move it or lose it' principle.

Our soft tissues – tendons, ligaments and muscles – need to work through their range of movement to stay strong and supple. This, in turn, allows us to live in comfort and move with ease and do the things we love, be it dancing, running, rowing or weightlifting.

You are probably only too well aware of this need to move more and would love to rediscover that natural flexibility, but lack time and energy, or are just not sure where to start. Maybe you've tried yoga and found the spiritual element off-putting or the bendy pretzel poses unobtainable for normal bodies.

Perhaps you find static stretching dull (you're not the only one!) or avoid stretching altogether but struggle to touch your toes or are sometimes aware of a niggling ache around your lower back.

The answer could be a style of dynamic stretching that will entertain even the most stretch-averse! A more playful, active style based on the premise that us humans naturally enjoy flowing motion, be it salsa dancing, running or t'ai chi. A style in stark contrast to sitting still and holding a stretch while the seconds tick by; one that will also offer the regular movement that health professionals tell us is vital to offset the stressful demands of modern life on the mind and body.

Move packages this, in the form of easy-to-follow, pre-prepared sequences called 'Moves' that do all the thinking and planning for you. There are only six Moves and these form the core of the book, so the concept is simple: each Move highlights an anatomical area, from Unstick the Hips to Hamstring Releasing.

Less mobile and want a simplified version done with the support of a chair? Look up their more Gentle counterparts. Mastered these Moves? Then brave the Advanced versions. The fact that there are harder and easier versions allows for both progression and modification, and means they are open to everyone.

The idea is to work systematically through anatomical areas using functional but fun movements. These are not tied to one exercise discipline, but are a blend of techniques I feel fit the brief of improving movement ease and efficiency, as well as improving posture and strengthening the core.

We've taken some gym-inspired mobility drills, included the odd animal inspired movement, added a pinch of strength work and mixed in a few yoga flows. Yoga bunnies will spot some staple classic poses such as Cat Stretch and Downward Dog. Gym-goers might recognise a hip flexibility technique or two from working on their squat form in the weights room.

Health-wise, some of the benefits will be immediately apparent, particularly in terms of releasing tension from areas such as the shoulders, which are quick to tense up. Move uses gentle motion to maintain a healthy back. The days of bed rest for lower back pain are over; the NHS now recommends staying 'as active as possible' using walking, yoga or Pilates, not only as rehab but also 'prehab' to maintain mobility and strength. Movement, as they say, is medicine!

Aside from the physical side, there are also clear mental benefits to be gained from taking 'brain breaks' in the day, which research has shown can stimulate a flagging mind. Slow, mindful movement, especially when paired with conscious, deep breathing, can also create what psychologists call a state of 'flow'. Being immersed in this flow state, created by synchronising the breath with movement, is fantastic for calming a busy mind, so works well after a frantic day.

So, where do we go from here? Before you dive in, take the time to read the next few pages, which will explain how to squeeze the most out of these sequences. We'll also delve into the language of movement, and explore the numerous health benefits and the science behind this style of stretching movement. What's more, I'll explain how to select and combine the Moves to enjoy the best 'release' depending on where you feel the most 'stuck', and which Moves will give keep you strong and injury-free for running, rugby or rowing.

There's plenty to explore, so let's get twisting, balancing, rolling and reaching. The end goal is a strong, mobile body, but we can have a lot of fun along the way playing with this active form of stretching.

Ready ... set ... Move.

THE BENEFITS OF STRETCHING WITH MOVEMENT

We know we should do some form of stretching but may be somewhat hazy about exactly why. The answer is that the range of health benefits, particularly for this type of dynamic – or motion-based – stretching, are surprisingly wide and varied.

By marrying stretching with movement we can tick several pages of boxes in terms of physical health and mental well-being. Yes, there are the obvious physical benefits of staying supple and the reduction in aches and niggles that flows from this, but there are also additional physical gains to be had in terms of a stronger core and improved posture. We are also increasingly discovering that taking regular movement 'brain breaks' has a psychological effect, too, increasing blood flow and oxygen levels, which may give the brain a boost and help to reduce feelings of stress.

Let's break it down and take a closer look at some reasons to swap sedentary for active.

REASONS TO STRETCH WITH MOVEMENT

1. Improves mobility or 'the ability to move freely'
Mobility is defined as 'the ability to move, or be moved freely and easily'. To get the science bit over and done with, it's the degree to which a joint can move ('range of motion') before being restricted by the surrounding soft tissue, such as tendons, muscle and ligaments. It's a little different to flexibility which is how far a muscle can lengthen and is achieved through static stretching (although the two terms are often used interchangeably).

As we age, or if we are sedentary for prolonged periods, our natural joint range of motion can become restricted. We might feel stiffer but are also in danger of injury as our bodies don't move as naturally and smoothly as they should. Regular movement maintains mobility and helps keep niggles and aches, especially in prime spots like the lower back, at bay.

2. Offsets the desk job
The human body is designed to move frequently but this might be quite hard to explain to your boss when a work deadline is looming and you are doing star jumps or walking lunges around the office. Just take a break when you can and look for little opportunities to walk, stretch and move. Public Health England

recommends we take 150 minutes of 'moderate' exercise every week, but this can be done in 10-minute bouts, which is easier to incorporate into a busy day.

If you work from home there are no excuses; pick one of the six Move sequences from this book and roll around on the carpet for 10 minutes before logging back on. The lower back and hamstrings, in particular, will thank you, as they tend to tighten up if you are stuck in a seated position day after day. The extra blood flow and oxygen may also give the brain a boost and help those creative ideas to flow. In an article called *Exercise, Movement and the Brain* in *Psychology Today,* Kimerer LaMothe, Ph.D. states: 'bodily movement is a cue for the brain to wake up … there are decisions to make, opportunities to take, dangers to avoid and pleasures to pursue … it's time to come fully online.'

For the desk-bound there are a range of chair-based Moves in the Gentle section, focusing on the neck, shoulders and back.

3. Soothes a frazzled mind

Movement, especially if it's synchronised with deep breathing, is fantastic for calming the mind. We know this from practising Eastern traditions such as yoga and t'ai chi, which have a joint spiritual and physical philosophy. The psychologist Mihaly Csikszentmihalyi first coined the term 'flow' to describe activities in which we are fully immersed and focused, and explained that yoga has many similarities to this state of flow. The mind can latch on to simple motion, especially if repeated a few times, and this allows it to concentrate (and stop overthinking). The awareness of breathing just makes the movement more mindful and less robotic, or mechanical, and forges a mind–body connection. In this way, we can take the Moves to another level. They can be done purely for the joy of movement, to maintain mobility and as a tool to calm the mind.

4. Makes you walk taller

Modern life demands that we spend a fair amount of time in a slightly flexed, or rounded-backed, position as we crunch numbers, pore over emails or fire out texts. Your body is often crying out, therefore, to 'open' or 'extend' by drawing back the shoulders and lifting the chest to redress this imbalance. The Lunge Flow and Shoulder Flossing Moves are particularly focused on improving posture, helping you sit, stand and walk taller. By following your schoolteacher's advice of 'stand up straight, shoulders back!' we can return the body to proper alignment. When the body is aligned correctly, with the head stacked above the shoulders (and not slumped down to create what physical therapists dub 'text neck') the strain, particularly on the lower and upper back, can be dramatically reduced.

5. Ensures your hammies play ball
If you love running, you'll want to run come rain or shine. It's the same with rowing, cycling or football. It's your stress buster and headspace time and the endorphins are amazing. So, you want your hamstrings, and other key muscles, to oblige and make the magic happen. Dynamic stretching drills are perfect for prepping the body for sport by warming up muscles, and gently increasing body temperature and heart rate, but they can also double up as cool-down stretches after sport if you don't like static stretching. The balancing techniques in the Main and Advanced Hamstring Releasing Move will also strengthen the muscles of the feet and ankles, and reinforce the core, which is a bonus for any sport that requires sprinting, running or jumping.

6. Is medicine for sore lower backs, necks, shoulders…
The hashtags 'movement is medicine' and 'motion is lotion' sum up the soothing nature of movement and why we always feel looser and less achy after a walk or run. The World Health Organisation estimates that 60–70 per cent of people living in industrialised countries will have 'non-specific' lower back pain, making it an extremely common problem. In the old days, 'bed rest' was the advice given, but health professionals now tend to favour gentle movement for the back muscles. Of course, the description 'back pain' is very vague and varies hugely from person to person. Check with your health professional that you have the all-clear to practise simple movements. If the answer is 'yes' then start with the Back Mobility Move sequence in the Gentle section of this book. There is the added attraction that it can be done while still lying in a nice, warm bed...

7. Keeps us young
Muscles can become stiffer with age, as do the supporting ligaments and tendons. There is also less synovial fluid – the lubricating liquid that envelops our joints and reduces friction. Dr Mark S. Lachs, Director of the Center for Aging Research at the Weill Medical College of Cornell University, recommends stretching and other gentle activity to encourage this fluid to become less viscous and flow more easily, thereby aiding and increasing movement. 'An analogy is [that of] applying a drop of oil to a stubborn gate and then opening and closing it until it stops squeaking', explains Lachs.

Often, people stop moving so much because they feel stiff and end up being even stiffer as they are moving less – it becomes a vicious cycle. So, try to incorporate a bit of motion every day. The Moves use repetitive motion ('reps') to maintain and improve mobility, and there are plenty of chair-based sequences in the Gentle section to choose from if kneeling on the floor doesn't appeal.

MOVEMENT SNACKING

If you have trouble dedicating a special time to 'exercise' once or twice a week then why not take the pressure off and try 'snacking' on movement throughout the day? Movement snacking simply means grabbing a few minutes of motion when you get a spare moment or in between tasks. No gym membership, special clothing or expensive equipment is required.

This idea of mini movement bouts is explored by Dr. Rangan Chatterjee in his book *The Four Pillar Plan*. Chatterjee states that small pockets of motion are more beneficial to health than sitting motionless for eight hours a day and then hitting the gym for 45 minutes of heart-pumping, high-intensity training.

So, what exactly constitutes a 'snack'? It could be squatting down to fill the washing machine, getting off the train a stop earlier and walking the rest of the way, balancing on one leg while cleaning your teeth, or sampling a sequence from this book. Humans are designed to move and our bodies love motion in multiple directions. This means not just folding forwards (which we do plenty of when sitting), but a regular mix of gentle back bending or 'extension', as well as rotating and stretching to the side, or 'lateral flexion'. Each Move routine in this book houses *all* of these types of movement so, in keeping with the dietary theme, they are like movement snacks – but laid out on a plate.

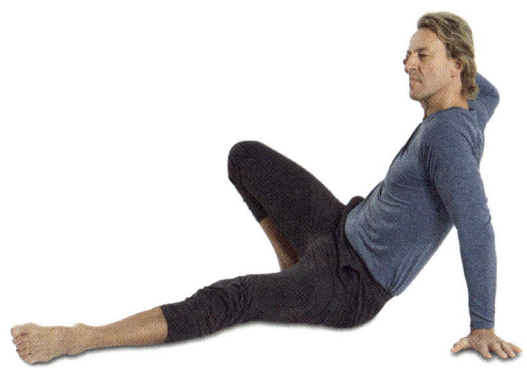

THE MOVE METHOD

Decoding the 'which, how and why' of stretching can be a tricky business, but this book is structured to take the guesswork out of staying supple. We've done all the thinking, selecting and planning for you, and produced six pre-packaged sequences or 'Moves'. Here's a simple guide to the Move method.

It's easy to hand-pick stretches from the vast range of sources out there but it's a tougher challenge to understand how to fuse them together in a routine that works logically through your hips, hamstrings or back. Move routines are pre-packaged so you don't have to do the thinking.

There are six ready-made sequences or Moves that comprise the core of the book, and each Move houses six techniques that work through a region of the body, releasing tension and promoting movement. However, because hips, backs or shoulders can't be neatly compartmentalised, but are interconnected, each Move strays into neighbouring regions. So, the Back Mobility Move, for instance, focuses on the back but also incorporates the shoulders and expands to include the front of the hips.

Although these six Moves are central, there are also both softer and more challenging versions of each. Mastered the basic Back Mobility Move? Then be brave and try the harder version in the Advanced section of this book. If you are low on energy, turn to Gentle Back Mobility.

Here's the low-down on your six Moves:

- Moves are ready-made sequences. They use an active, flowing style of stretching based on exploring and increasing joint range of motion. A movement is repeated using 'reps' to gradually loosen up an area, resulting in improved mobility.

- There are six Moves. Each Move houses six techniques. These six Main Moves form the core of the book, but there are harder versions in the Advanced section and easier ones in the Gentle section.

- Pick one Move, or link all six together. A single Move takes roughly five minutes so it would take 30 minutes to complete all six. Woken up with a stiff back but feeling lazy? Lie back and do the Back Mobility Move while still in bed. There is no timetable or programme – it depends on the time and energy you have available.

- Moves highlight an anatomical area. This area may be the hips, back, hamstrings and shoulders, but it could stray into other interconnected regions, making the Move an effective whole-body mobility routine in itself. The human body can't be cleanly mapped and carved into neat sections like a diagram of beef cuts! The culprit causing all the trouble in your hips might be a nearby lower back muscle. The Moves are designed to take this into account.

- Moves do *all* the moves. The body needs to be eased through all the main planes of motion to reduce strain and maintain balance. These are flexion (forward bending), extension (back bending), rotation (twisting) and lateral flexion (side bending). These terms describe the actions of the spine in the movement.

- Stay standing, sitting or lying. Each Move sticks to one body position – lying, standing, sitting or all fours – so you don't need to constantly shift position. This means that one technique slides seamlessly into the next, creating a nice feeling of flow.

- No kit is required. Moves require no equipment, simply a floor space (or a chair if you are doing some of the chair-based Gentle versions) that's big enough for you to lunge or roll around in without colliding with the dog.

- Move day or night. Moves can be practised at any time of the day, but as muscles feel stiffer in the morning, that's the time to ease in gently with a Move to warm up your body; Back Mobility would do this nicely. Research has shown that our muscles reach peak pliability in the afternoon so that's the time to ramp things up and brave an Advanced sequence. Finally, most of the Moves work last thing at night, but slow the speed and synchronise your breathing with the movement for a more chilled-out effect.

- Go easy on yourself. Nothing in the Moves should hurt! The idea is to slide in and out of the movements smoothly five or six times (the 'reps') but on each rep only come to the edge of the full stretch. So, stop short of your maximum range of motion and certainly never push to the point of pain. Also, if you have a medical condition or are new to exercise, check with your medical practitioner that you are good to go.

- Don't forget to play. Last but not least, find your inner kid! The Moves are designed to be playful, exploring techniques such as Side Sweeps, Rolling Bridges, Kite Flying and Shoulder Flossing. You are also encouraged to rip up the rulebook and experiment with variations of the movements. Look for the Play sign dotted throughout the Moves, which offers suggestions.

MOVE IT OR LOSE IT

Flexibility is joint-specific. That means you might not be able bend over easily to tie your shoelaces (poor hamstring/lower back flexibility) but can easily apply sun cream to that tricky space between your shoulder blades without asking for help (superior shoulder flexibility). Technically, therefore, there's no such thing as an 'inflexible' person, just joints that are more, or less, supple.

Joint mobility is assessed using the lovely-sounding 'degrees of freedom'. The ball-and-socket shoulder joint has the most degrees of freedom as we can do pretty much any movement with it, from reaching up to a high shelf (flexion) to spinning it in circles like a bowler in cricket (circumduction). This makes the shoulder the most mobile joint in the body. However, a tightening of muscle and thickening of fascia – the connective tissue layer just under the skin – can, over time, impede even this highly flexible joint.

The influence of fascia on flexibility is currently being studied but some believe it can become thicker in certain parts of the body and this creates rigidity or stiffness. Alternatively, fascia can become knotted through repetitive movements in sport. This not only prevents our shoulders from moving as nature intended, but can also lead to tension and pain.

Dynamic stretching is a fantastic way to loosen fascia and help us to retain our natural freedom of movement and avoid strain. We are not trying to sit cross-legged in a full Lotus position, just enjoy tension-free, wide-ranging movement.

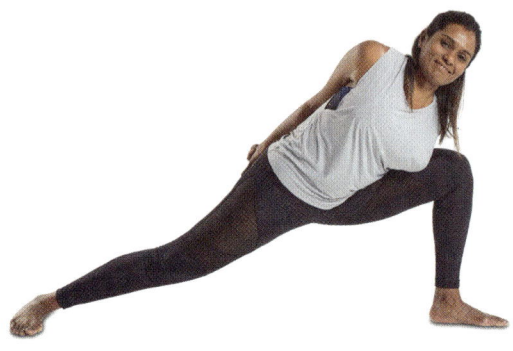

WHICH MOVE TO CHOOSE?

Which Moves you choose depends on where you need to be loosened up the most. Here are a few suggestions for how to liberate your tightest spots. What do we want? Physical freedom! When do we want it? Now!

For many, the shoulders or lower back are first on any 'stiff list'. This will certainly be the case if your work involves slaving over a desk or laptop. But hamstrings come a pretty close second, particularly if you do a lot of sport. Don't worry – if you feel sore or restricted in these common areas, or any of following tight spots, there's salvation to be had. I've recommended a few Move sequences, hand-picked from the Main, Gentle and Advanced sections of this book, to free up your body.

Stiff lower back – Back Mobility (Gentle and Main), Cat Play (Gentle and Main) and Lunge Flow (Gentle and Main)

Achy shoulders – Cat Play (Gentle and Main) and Shoulder Flossing (Gentle and Main)

Tight hamstrings – Hamstring Releasing (Gentle) and Lunge Flow (Gentle and Main)

Poor balance – Hamstring Releasing (Main and Advanced)

Improved posture – Lunge Flow (Main and Advanced) and Shoulder Flossing (Main and Advanced)

Tight hip flexors and quadriceps (anterior hip and thigh) – Lunge Flow (Gentle, Main and Advanced)

Tight gluteals (buttocks) – Unstick the Hips (Gentle, Main and Advanced) and Lunge Flow (Gentle, Main and Advanced)

As you can see, I've only picked two or three Moves, but if you have time to do all six please do; you'll leave the whole body feeling super-stretched and tingly. If you never suffer with any stiff bits just keep moving, stretching and doing what you're doing to stay ache-free, and enjoy any one of the Moves.

MOVES USE DYNAMIC STRETCHING

The type of stretching we are working with is classified as 'dynamic'. This essentially means stretching with movement. This type of stretching warms up the synovial fluid that lubricates our joints to facilitate better movement. Athletes use it both as a warm-up to get the blood pumping and as a cool-down to aid venous blood return to the heart. Because of this circulatory aspect you may feel a little more awake and energised, which means these sequences are fantastic to perform first thing in the morning. In flexibility terms, dynamic stretching is great for improving joint range of motion, which is the full movement potential of a joint. In plain language, we are exploring movement to encourage the body to function as it was designed to — with maximum ease and minimum restriction.

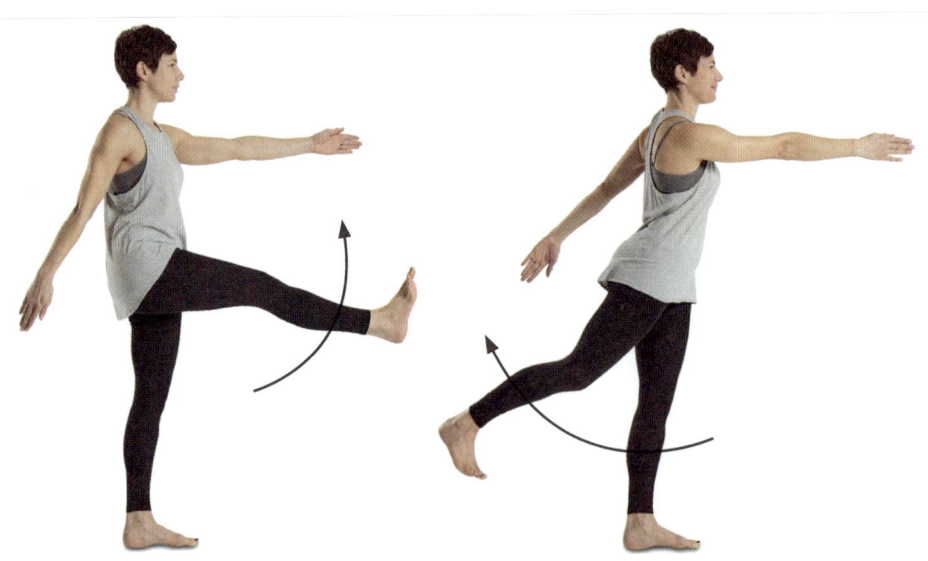

MOVE RULES

The word 'rules' seems out of place in a book about breaking free and exploring movement, but these four will keep you safe and ensure you gain the most from your Move experience.

MOVE SLOWLY
Muscles react to fast, jerky movements by contracting. It's called the myotatic, or stretch, reflex and is a nervous system response to protect from injury a muscle the body feels is lengthening too quickly. Slow stretching, accompanied by deep breathing through the nose, will dull these signals and allow the joints to move through their full range with less restriction. Moving slowly is also a more mindful way of moving, so switching to slo-mo has both a neurological and psychological effect.

STRETCH WITH WARM MUSCLES
It is possible to pull muscles when stretching, particularly first thing in the morning when they are not sufficiently warmed up, so don't stretch in a cold or draughty place. Warm muscles are also more pliable and responsive to stretching.

PRACTISE LITTLE AND OFTEN
If you want to see improvements in flexibility, 'little and often' will reap rewards. So, stretching three times a week for five minutes each time is better than a single 20-minute session once a week.

LISTEN TO YOUR BODY
The Main Moves are designed to suit as many bodies as possible, but only you know yourself, so if you have an old shoulder injury or lower back problems go gently and never push a stretch beyond a comfortable range. If you have a very tight area that is not releasing through this type of dynamic stretching, try holding the stretch statically for 30–40 seconds.

HOW TO BREATHE

If you've never done yoga or Pilates before you may be thinking 'I know how to breathe!' But pairing movement with breathing makes both physiological and psychological sense so it's well worth mastering the basics.

Breathing combined with movement is used by systems such as yoga to create a feeling a 'flow', which calms and focuses the mind. It also benefits the mechanical process of stretching by affecting the nervous system so that we can fold, rotate or dip a little deeper. So, let's run through the benefits of breathing and play with a few simple techniques. Ready? Inhale ... and exhale.

There are reasons why all the Move instructions in this book contain cues for when to breathe, the main one being to make the exercises feel more mindful and less robotic or mechanical. By timing the movement with the breath we involve the mind and so the techniques are transformed from the purely physical – 'raise your left arm up' – to much more of a combined mind–body experience. It also forces you to slow down the movement as you have to wait until you are ready to breathe in or out before you move. This is nice if, like most people, you rush through the day ticking off tasks and need a slower pace.

If you've done dynamic, or flowing, styles of yoga before then I'm preaching to the converted. If all this talk of breathing is new to you, don't worry, the instructions tell you exactly when to inhale and exhale. However, generally, you inhale in the start position – let's call it A – and exhale into the final position or B.

Breathe in and out through your nose, rather than your mouth; the nasal passages are narrow, so this helps to slow down the breathing pace. It also just feels more relaxing than oral breathing.

What's more, there's another reason why deeper breathing is great paired with movement and it's to do with our nervous system. When we breathe deeply it helps to switch off the sensory receptors or 'muscle spindles' that tell muscles to contract if we stretch too fast or far (the same myotatic response mentioned earlier). This allows muscles to lengthen more, which lets us fold, extend or rotate deeper. This is especially helpful with static stretching; for example, the lunge position that is held throughout the Lunge Flow Move.

This 'moving with the breath' business can take a bit of getting used to. However, if you're wondering 'do I inhale here?', be reassured that at some point it just 'clicks', and feels a normal and natural part of conscious movement.

NOTICE, COUNT AND FLOW: THREE STEPS TO MOVING WITH YOUR BREATH

If linking movement with breathing is new to you, try these three simple techniques. The first is a tuning-in exercise, the second focuses on breathing deeper, and the third practises synchronising the breath and movement.

NOTICE
Just sit with a straight back and relax your shoulders. Close your eyes and breathe in and out through your nose. Visualise the air flowing through both nostrils and start to lengthen both the inhalation and exhalation a touch so that you are breathing a little bit deeper than you normally would. Take 10 of these deeper breaths.

COUNT
Now count your inhalation and exhalation so that you breathe in for a count of one, two, three, four and breathe out for a count of one, two, three, four. If this feels too short, count up to five or six seconds, but don't strain to get there; you should be comfortably reaching a higher count.

FLOW
Finally, get accustomed to moving with the breath by synchronising your breathing with a simple action, such as raising both arms above your head. Inhale to raise the arms up and exhale to return them down. Practise timing it so you finish the inhalation when your arms are at their highest point and the exhalation comes to an end just as your arms reach your sides. Repeat this four–six times.

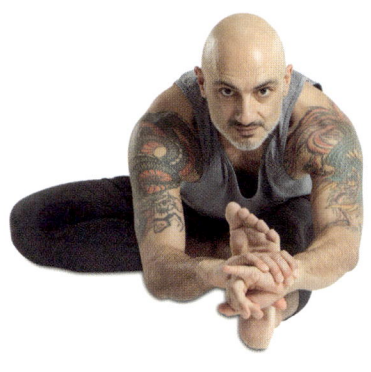

THE LANGUAGE OF MOVEMENT

The following words and phrases pop up in this book to describe movement. Some are official anatomical terms while others you might hear in a yoga or Pilates class. Here's the low-down on the language of movement.

Flexion – An anatomical term to describe any movement that decreases the angle between two bones, e.g. bending the arm at the elbow brings the forearm closer to the upper arm. It is commonly used in this book to describe the action of raising the arms above the head but we also often 'flex' the spine or curl it into a rounded position.

Extension – The anatomical word for any movement that increases the angle between two bones, e.g. straightening the arm at the elbow takes the forearm further away from the upper arm. It is used in this book to describe the action of reaching the arms behind you when standing. We also often 'extend' the spine by arching the back, or performing what would be called a 'back bend' in gymnastics. Flexion and extension are often used together, e.g. alternately flexing and extending the spine to mobilise the back. This technique is used repeatedly in the Cat Play Move.

Rotation – Any movement that involves a twisting action of the body – usually originating from the torso, e.g. turning to look over your shoulder. Rotations or 'twists' in this book are done standing, on all fours, sitting and lying.

Lateral flexion – In a yoga class this would be called 'side bending'. It simply describes a movement where the body tips not forwards or back but to the side. We use it to stretch the sides of the body, especially the hips and outer thigh. It is not a movement naturally done in everyday life, but is especially useful for people who do sports such as running and cycling, which focus on forwards-only movement.

Engage the core – This is an instruction to brace the muscles that wrap around the torso in order to create a more stable midsection. It is used in this book to help prevent overloading the lower back muscles when exiting positions bending forward, or in preparation for core strengthening work. Rather than suck the belly in try placing your hands on your middle and cough sharply. You will feel your core muscles momentarily 'switch on'. Repeat this a few times until you learn how it should feel when you consciously engage the core.

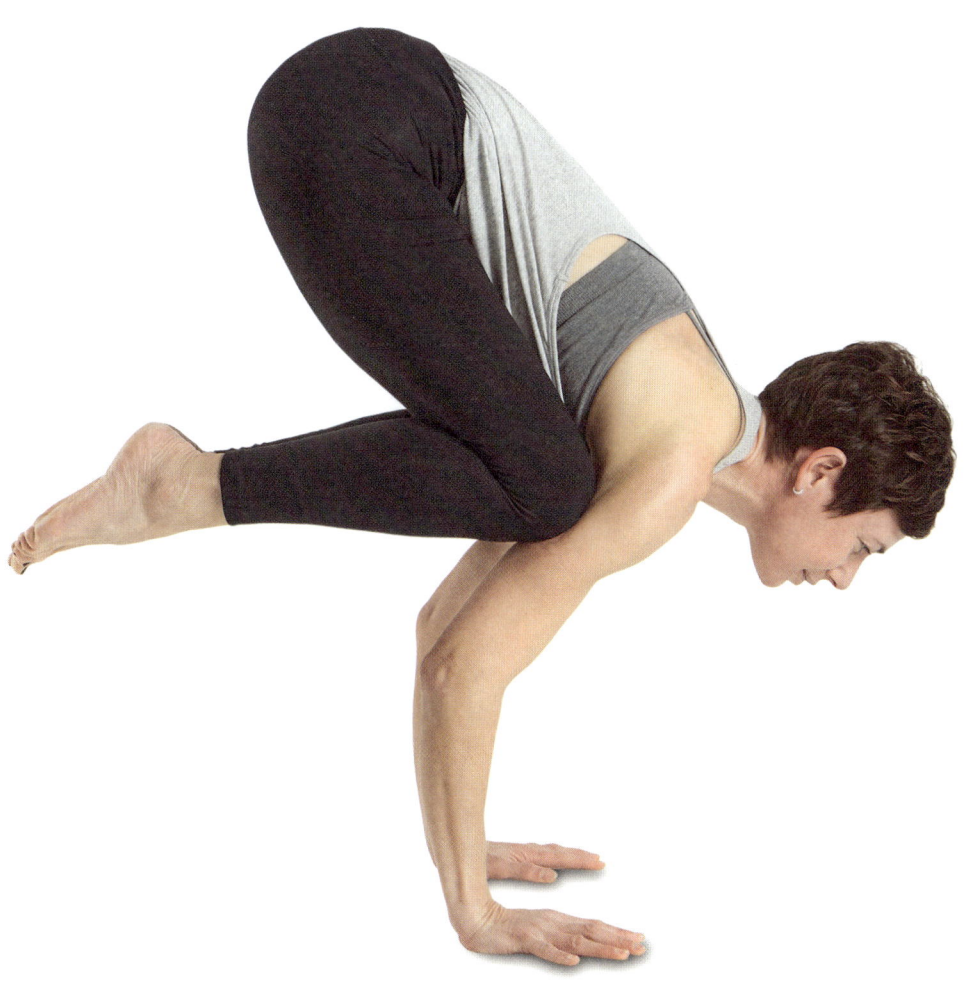

MOVES AND SPORT

Love sport but hate to stretch? A more active, energetic style of stretching could be the answer to staying injury-free (and entertained).

If you find yourself skipping post-exercise stretching in favour of the shower or protein shake, but realise the value of maintaining flexibility in terms of both injury prevention and performance, dynamic stretching can be a fun alternative to holding a stretch and counting the seconds.

Let's start with some definitions: 'dynamic stretching' is any stretch involving movement, including the techniques in our Move sequences. A stretch is 'static' if it is held still, usually for 10–20 seconds. Static stretching is very useful for increasing flexibility but is seen as dull by many athletes, maybe because this stillness contrasts starkly with the active sports they love.

In an ideal world we should do a bit of both: dynamic stretching to warm up pre-sport and static stretching afterwards (deep static stretching done before sport has been shown to reduce power). However, if you're neglecting stretching completely and need to take action, the dynamic option will tick a lot of boxes in terms of maintaining mobility (and keeping you engaged and entertained).

Maintaining the body's natural movement is crucial as most sports can gradually erode range of movement over time. This especially applies to running, hiking and cycling where we move repetitively within a limited range. For example, in cycling the legs remain slightly bent so the hamstrings never fully lengthen.

Combine this limited range of sporting movement with a day job that involves the legs and hips remaining flexed all day while you sit at a desk and we can see the need for remedial movement.

These sports also move within what is called the 'sagittal' or 'front to back' plane, so it's important to break out and explore other directions, such as rotational movements (frontal plane) and lateral or side-to-side movements (also the frontal plane), both of which the Moves offer.

What's more, the Moves can also enhance performance for sports. This might be increasing the range of a golf swing or enabling you to go deeper into a squat for weightlifting, and they can aid sports that require excellent upper body flexibility, such as swimming. Think of them as mobility drills.

So, when should you use the Moves for sport? They work well both as a warm-up to prep muscles and tendons, and a cool-down while the heart rate returns to normal – the gentle movement acts as a muscle pump, aiding venous blood flow back to the heart.

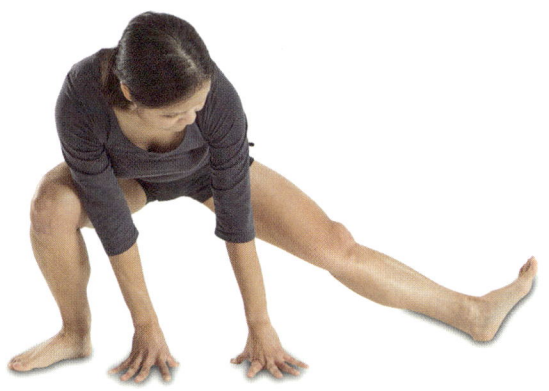

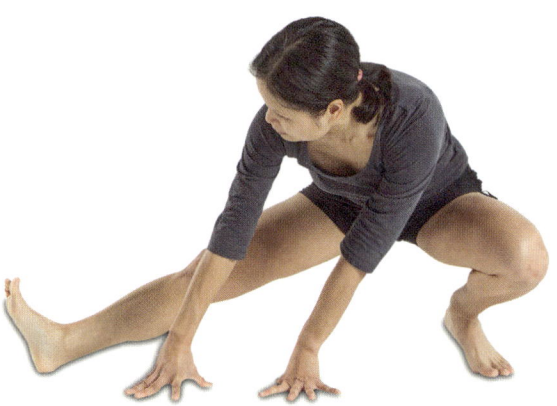

However, it is important to stress that static stretching has a valuable place in maintaining flexibility in sport, too. It is especially recommended if you have a very tight area. This level of restriction may either impact performance or lead to injury as the body can't move as it should. My suggestion in these cases would be to use the Moves to really warm up the area, then just pause the sequence and hold. There are several invitations to do this in the instructions.

WHICH MOVE TO CHOOSE FOR SPORT

If you're keen to try a Move but are unsure which is the best match for your running, rugby or rowing body, here are a few combinations that will work wonders.

The Move sequences are very versatile for sport. As discussed, they can be used as both warm-up and cool-down sequences, but also in between matches, runs or rides to maintain mobility. The list below is not definitive, so feel free to sample any of the Moves; I have picked the ones I feel best target the tightest spots for each sport.

In some cases I've mixed in Advanced or Gentle versions of the Moves. For example, if you are a serious swimmer then you can really improve your upper body range of motion by trying to do all three Shoulder Flossing sequences (Gentle first, then Main and Advanced). It's still important to work within your flexibility limits, never pushing to the point of pain. If you're feeling stiff, or are injured, stick to the Gentle Moves until you are strong and ready to progress.

Baseball and softball – Lunge Flow (Main and Advanced) and Shoulder Flossing (Main and Advanced)

Basketball and netball – Lunge Flow (Main), Shoulder Flossing (Main) and Hamstring Releasing (Main and Advanced)

Cycling – Cat Play (Gentle and Main), Unstick the Hips (Gentle and Main) and Shoulder Flossing (Gentle and Main)

Golf – Back Mobility (Gentle and Main), Cat Play (Gentle and Main) and Shoulder Flossing (Main and Advanced)

Hiking and walking – Back Mobility (Gentle and Main) and Hamstring Releasing (Gentle and Main)

Hockey (ice and field) – Back Mobility (Gentle and Main), Lunge Flow (Main) and Hamstring Releasing (Main and Advanced)

Rowing – Back Mobility (Gentle and Main), Hamstring Releasing (Gentle) and Cat Play (Main)

Rugby – Cat Play (Gentle and Main), Lunge Flow (Main) and Shoulder Flossing (Gentle and Main)

Running – Hamstring Releasing (Gentle, Main and Advanced), Unstick the Hips (Main and Advanced) and Lunge Flow (Main and Advanced)

Soccer – Hamstring Releasing (Gentle, Main and Advanced), Unstick the Hips (Gentle and Main) and Lunge Flow (Gentle and Main)

Swimming – Cat Play (Main) and Shoulder Flossing (Main and Advanced)

Triathlon – Hamstring Releasing (Gentle and Main), Unstick the Hips (Main), Lunge Flow (Gentle and Main) and Shoulder Flossing (Main)

Weight training – Cat Play (Main), Unstick the Hips (Main and Advanced) and Shoulder Flossing (Gentle and Main)

Tennis – Hamstring Releasing (Main and Advanced), Lunge Flow (Main) and Shoulder Flossing (Main and Advanced)

As you can see, I have only suggested two or three Moves for each sport but you could also explore others or work through all six, from Back Mobility all the way to Shoulder Flossing. Since each sequence takes only five minutes, this means that all six will be done and dusted in 30 minutes. That's just half an hour to complete a comprehensive head-to-toe mobility session that will keep you strong and supple for the sports you love.

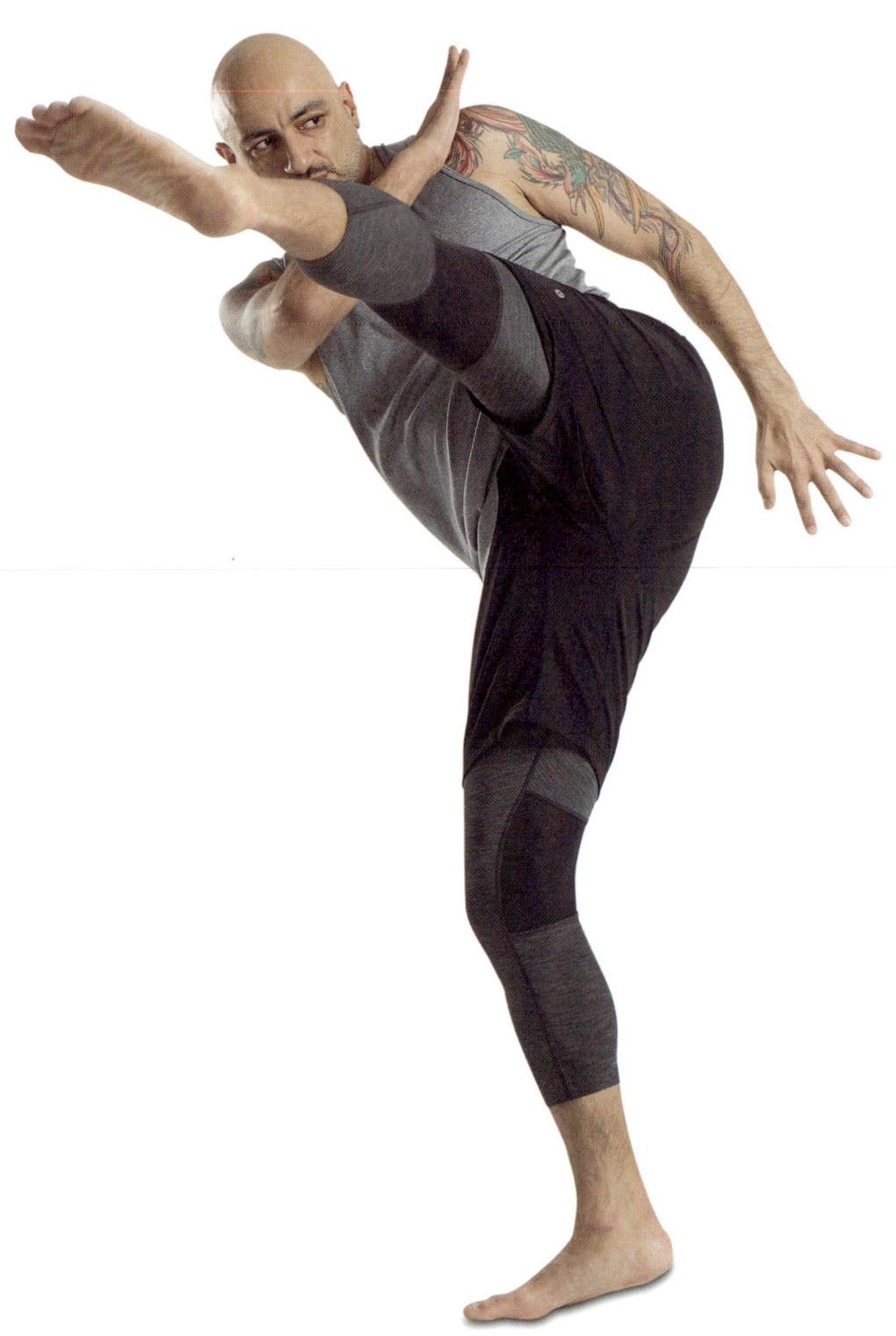

TESTIMONIALS

Here's what people who do just five minutes of Moves per day have to say about how it makes them feel.

'Ten feet tall!'
Rachel, *human resources director*

'Less stiff and sore and more mobile; stretching helps me loosen up key muscle groups, improve mobility, and I'm convinced it prevents injuries and aids faster recovering after training.'
Adam, *triathlete*

'Like I've been unravelled! I spend all day at my desk and then pretty much every sport I do, like boxing and cycling, I'm hunching my shoulders. I want to do something about my posture before I get older and it's harder to remedy.'
James, *advertising executive*

'Calm, strong, grounded and content with the world and myself.'
Susannah, *barrister*

'It allows me to spread out when I've been sitting studying in the same position for a long time. My body wants to move. It's almost involuntary, my knee starts twitching and I have to get up and stretch.'
Ollie, *student*

'A lot freer! My golf swing has improved dramatically since I started because my upper body flexibility has changed so much.'
John, *retired*

'Better! It sorts out all the wonkiness and releases my "granny hips" and super-tight back. I started out as a converted sceptic and am now a passionate mover!'
Isabelle, *teacher*

'More robust physically and mentally so I'm ready to live my best life.'
Julia, *architect*

Starting the journey to a stronger, happier body couldn't be simpler. The six Moves are waiting… So good luck and enjoy.

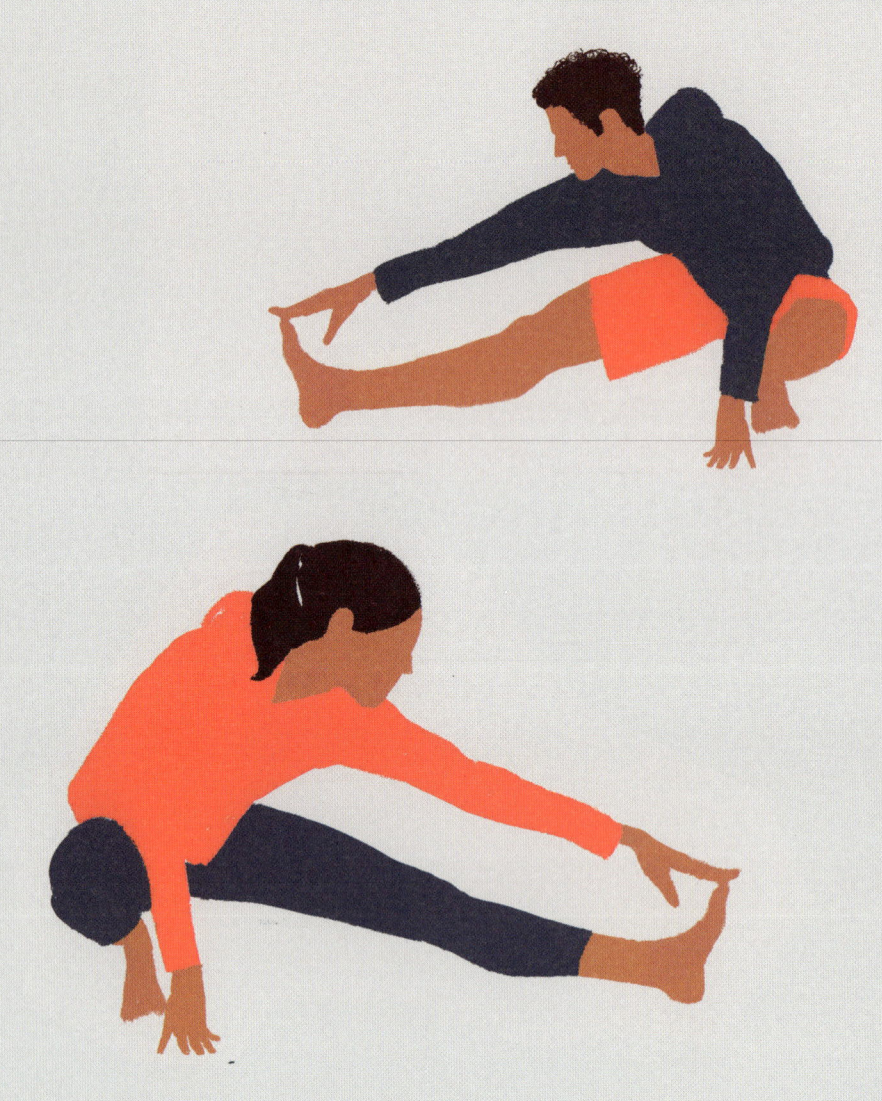

THE MOVES

So here they are, the six sequences or 'Moves' that form the core of this book.

Moves are a hand-picked selection of movements designed to improve mobility, using a fun, active and flowing style of stretching to systematically loosen up a specific area, from the hips and hamstrings up to the neck and shoulders. These pre-packed sequences contain a dose of dynamic stretches, a pinch of flow yoga, a few mobility drills borrowed from the gym boys and girls, and a dash of strength and balance.

TARGETED

Each Move targets a specific anatomical area. There are two Moves for the back, two for the hips, one for the hamstrings and one for the shoulders. However, the sequences often stray beyond these anatomical borders to become whole-body mobility exercises.

FLOW-ABLE

Each Move sticks to one position, such as sitting, lunging or standing, which means that you are not constantly shifting up and down to the floor. This consistency allows you to flow more easily from one technique to the next with minimal disruption.

GO HARD ... OR EASE OFF

These six Moves are the Main sequences of the book, but we also offer Gentle and Advanced versions of all of them. These easier and harder versions mirror the Main Moves closely. This makes it easier to progress from Gentle to Main, or Main to Advanced.

PICK AND MIX

Moves are pretty versatile! The easiest option is simply to do them in order, from one to six. This will take around 30 minutes and leave the entire body feeling stretched, aligned and revitalised – a whole-body reboot! If you are short of time just select the Move that suits you best. You can also mix in techniques from Advanced and Gentle versions to create your own tailor-made sequence.

GET CREATIVE

You will spot the odd 'Play' sign scattered through the Moves. This is an invitation to explore variations of the movements. Feel free to sample these, or wander off script altogether and concoct your own.

Moves will help regain that natural freedom of movement for which our bodies were designed. A body that moves like this, without restraint, is less resistant to everyday aches and niggles, and simply feels fantastic. So let's get moving!

MOVE 1
BACK MOBILITY

Don't stagger robot-like out of bed when the alarm goes off, savour a few minutes more and ease into the day with these limbering-up movements designed to make you feel a little less mechanical and a little more human. This first sequence introduces techniques for a happy, healthy back, leaving you warmed up and primed to go.

The spine is like the frame or chassis of your body and provides the foundation for better movement, so it makes sense for us to begin with the back, particularly if you've ever complained of a tight, stiff or even sore back, neck or shoulders.

By starting lying face up (supine) we can not only stay in bed a little longer, but also assess which back zones move well, and which feel tight or restricted, without any strain. This is particularly useful if you are taking special care of your lower back, although this position provides a great entry point into movement exploration for everyone and is recommended as step one of the six Moves.

So, first we'll mobilise the spine and release the lower back. Then we'll venture further up to explore the mid-back, or thoracic spine – for many the stiffest part of the back – before arriving at the upper back and shoulders.

Think of this first Move, therefore, as a 'checking in' sequence before expanding down to the hips and legs and branching out to the shoulders in later Moves. By easing the spine into gentle flexion (hugging the legs in), extension (lifting the hips into bridge) and rotation (swaying the knees from side to side) we can tick off the key movements that a happy, healthy back requires.

Rolling Bridges is an exercise in connecting with your spine. The idea is to visualise it less as a single solid 'back bone' and more as a highly movable structure that you can begin to isolate and segment. As you roll up and down, imagine your spine as a string of pearls or bicycle chain and lift up/lay down each vertebra one at a time. If this is too tricky, start by dividing the back into three sections: 1) lower back, 2) mid-back and 3) shoulder blades. As you roll up, lift the lower back, then the mid-back, then the shoulder blades and reverse this as you roll down, deliberately pressing each section down into the floor one at a time.

STEP 1

LOWER BACK MASSAGE

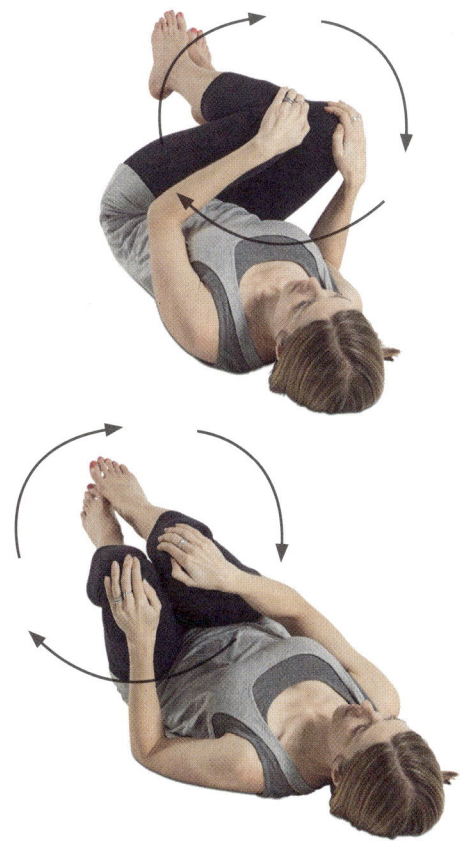

- Lie on your back with your legs bent.
- Hug both legs into your belly.
- Place one hand on each knee.
- Keeping your knees together, move them in slow circles to massage the lower back.
- Breathe in and out as you massage.

REPS:
Four–six circles.

MOVE 1: Back Mobility

STEP 2

ROLLING BRIDGES

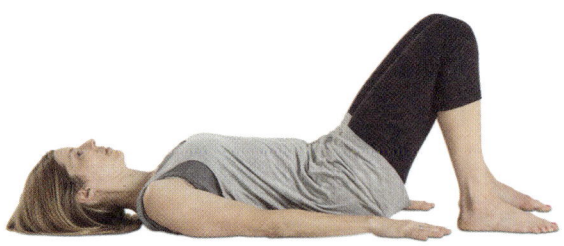

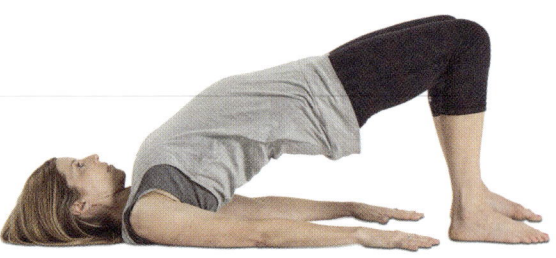

- Bend both legs and place your feet on the floor, hip-width apart.
- Place your arms by your sides, palms facing down.
- Press your lower back into the floor.
- Inhale and peel your hips off the ground, then your mid-back, then your shoulder blades until you are in the Bridge position.
- Exhale and reverse the movement by laying down your shoulder blades, mid-back and hips.
- Continue, inhaling to peel the spine up and exhaling to lay the spine down.

REPS: Six.

TIP: Visualise your spine as a highly mobile chain of smaller bones, rather than a solid single 'backbone'.

STEP 3

ALTERNATE LEG HUGS

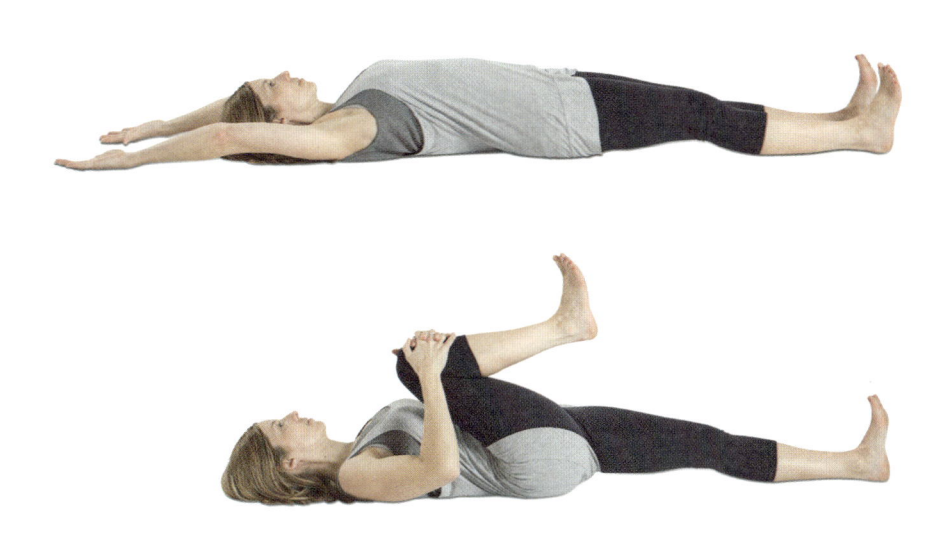

- Stretch your legs out straight with your toes pointing up.
- Place your arms by your sides, palms facing down.
- As you inhale, sweep both arms above your head.
- As you exhale, hug your right leg into your body.
- Inhale and sweep both arms above your head as you return your right leg to the floor.
- Exhale and hug your left leg into your body.
- Inhale and sweep both arms above your head as you return your left leg to the floor.
- Repeat, moving smoothly from leg to leg.

REPS: Four on each side.

STEP 4

THORACIC RELEASER

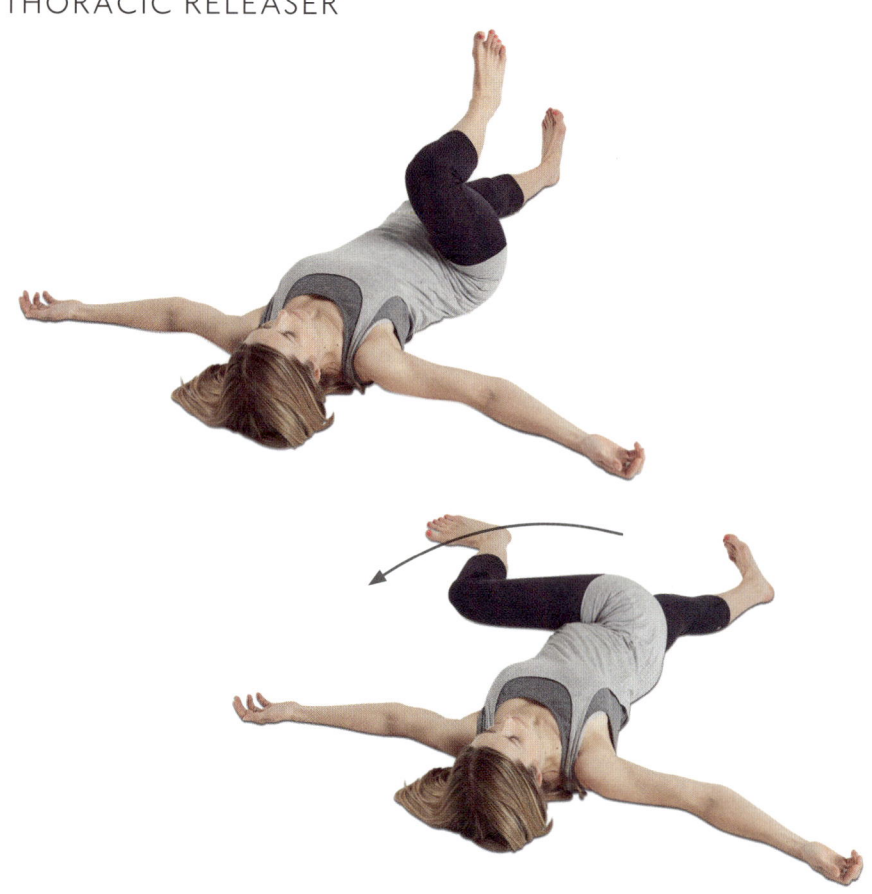

- Hug your right leg in and press your lower back slightly to the floor.
- Keeping your leg here, stretch your arms out at shoulder height, palms facing up.
- Inhale. As you exhale, swing the leg across the body to the left, keeping both shoulders grounded.
- Inhale and swing the leg back to the centre.
- Complete the reps.
- Switch sides by hugging the left leg in.

REPS: Four on each side.

STEP 5

BOOK PAGES

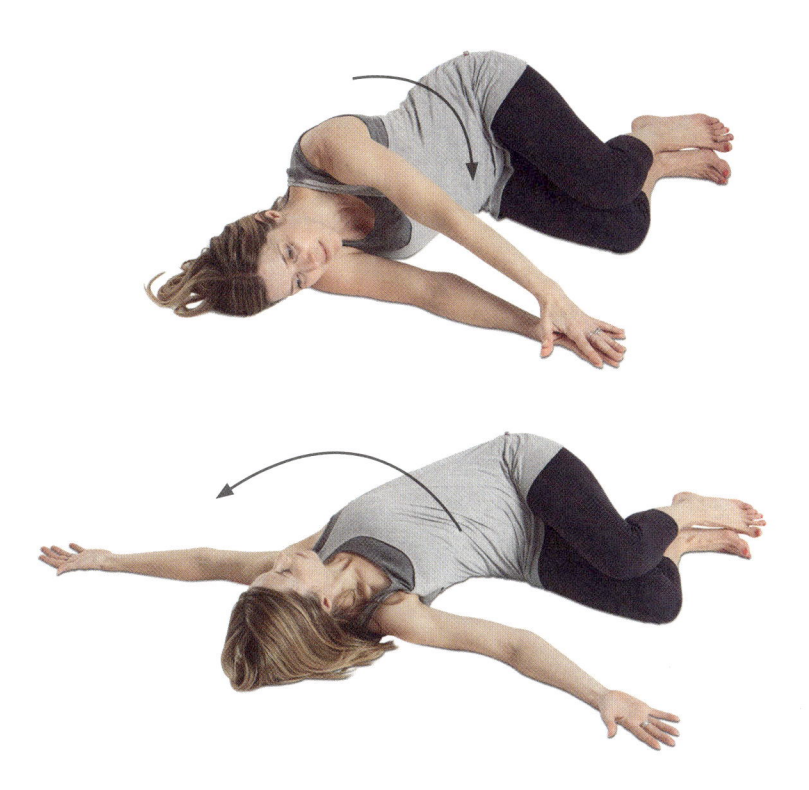

- Lie on your right side with your knees bent into a 90-degree angle.
- Straighten your arms and place your palms together.
- Inhale and sweep your left arm out to the left. It may hang suspended, or drop all the way to the floor.
- Exhale and return your arm to the starting position, placing your palms together.
- Continue opening and closing the arm for the specified number of reps.
- Roll on to your left side and repeat.

REPS: Four on each side.

PLAY: As you place your palms together, slide your top hand past your lower hand to stretch into the shoulder.

MOVE 1: Back Mobility

STEP 6

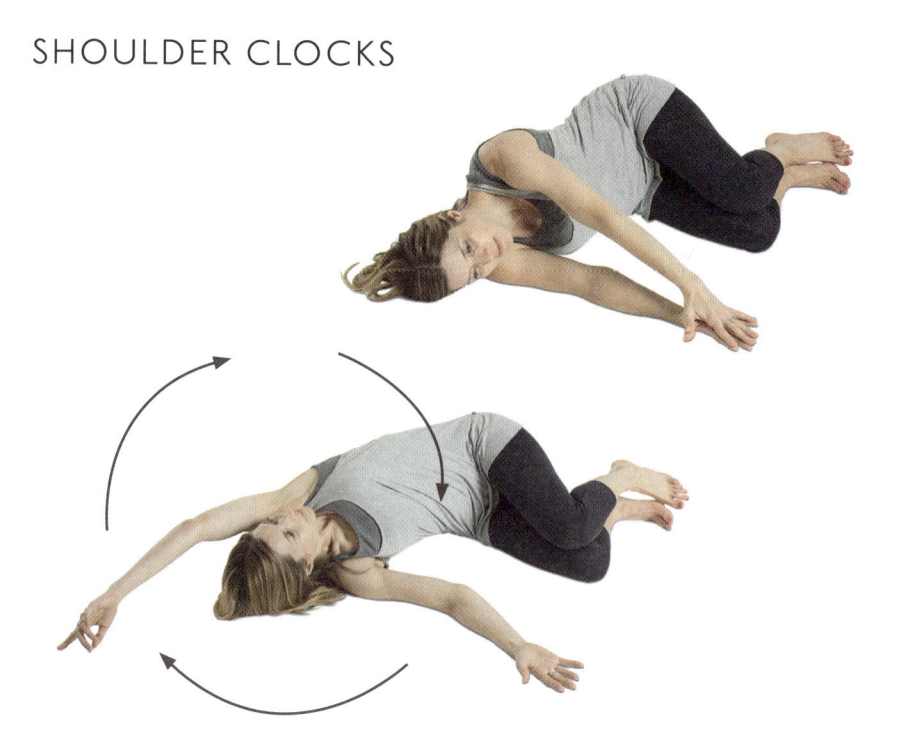

SHOULDER CLOCKS

- Roll on to your right side.
- Make a large circular sweeping movement with your left arm. Keep the breath flowing in and out as you circle.
- Make two circles clockwise and two anticlockwise. Work slowly, thinking about keeping your fingertips close to the floor.
- Complete the reps.
- Roll on to the left side and repeat.

REPS: Four on each side (two clockwise, two anticlockwise).

PLAY: Gradually work on circling with your fingertips closer to the floor.

CHANGE IT UP

If you want it tougher...
Try the Advanced version of this Move on page 132.

If you want it more gentle...
For a less-strenuous version of this Move, see page 86.

40 MOVE

MOVE 2
CAT PLAY

We take a cue from our furry friends and play with 'pandiculation' with this second sequence, which is packed with feline techniques to iron out any kinks in the back and shoulders, and promote fluid, tension-free movement. So get down on all fours, cat-like, and go searching for tight spots.

This all-fours sequence mimics the head-down/bottom-up stretch cats and dogs do to ease stiff, rigid limbs into movement after a deep sleep. The technical name for this yawn–stretch action is 'pandiculation' from the Latin 'to stretch oneself'.

Along with that famous yoga technique Cat Stretch, it is our inspiration for priming the back, shoulders and hips for more fluid, tension-free movement.

Cat Play is a step on from Move 1 Back Mobility as it introduces more range of motion in the back and shoulders by dipping, dropping and reaching further. Built around Cat Stretch, the technique guides the body through deeper flexion (forward bending), extension (back bending), side bending and rotation.

That back-arching extension movement is perhaps the most welcome and satisfying of all, especially if you've spent the day sitting with a slightly flexed spine and are itching to ease that into reverse by lifting the chest and drawing back the shoulders. Having said that, don't be tempted to push up too high into the deeper backbend Cobra (Cobra Flow) if you have any lower back issues. Staying low is a more gentle option and will avoid compressing that lumbar, or lower back, area.

Thoracic Twist targets the stiffest part of the back: the mid-back or thoracic zone. To ensure that you reach this spot effectively, keep your hips still and stay looking down to lock off the lower back and neck.

The final step – Freestyle Cat – involves a big element of play as you explore all these planes of motion in your own time. The purpose? To hunt out the tight spots where your back feels most restricted and ease out any stiffness through slow, mindful movement. So see what feels good: sit back on your heels, turn to peek over your shoulder or round the back. Rip up the rulebook and go with it.

STEP 1

CAT STRETCH

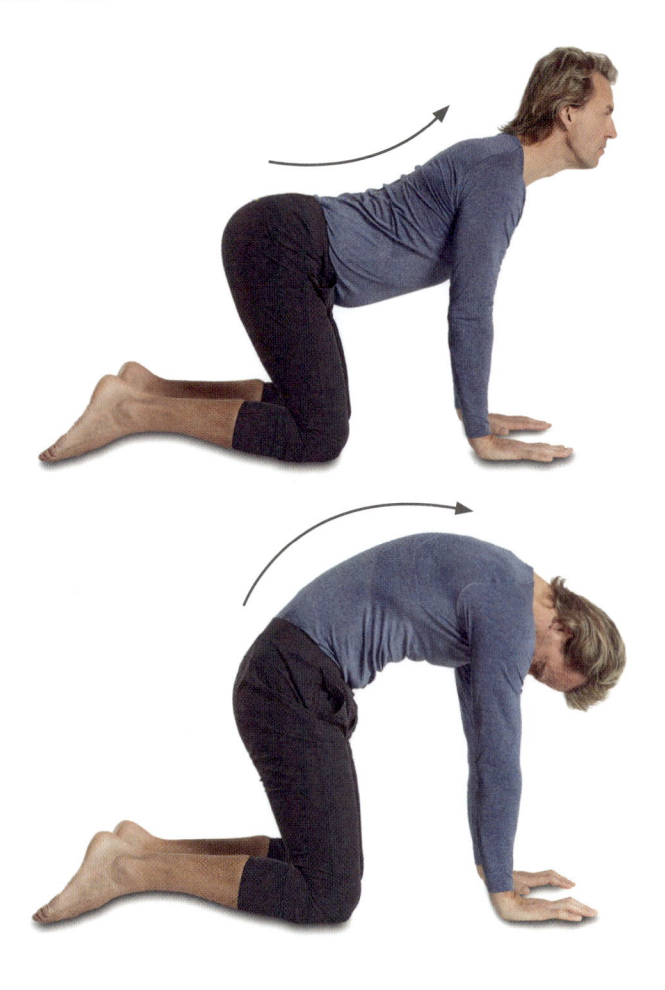

- Start on all fours.
- As you inhale, lift the head and hips, allowing the mid-back to dip.
- As you exhale, flex your back by lifting and rounding the spine, tucking your chin in towards your chest.
- Repeat, inhaling to lift and exhaling to round.

REPS: Six.

STEP 2

SIDE CRAWLING

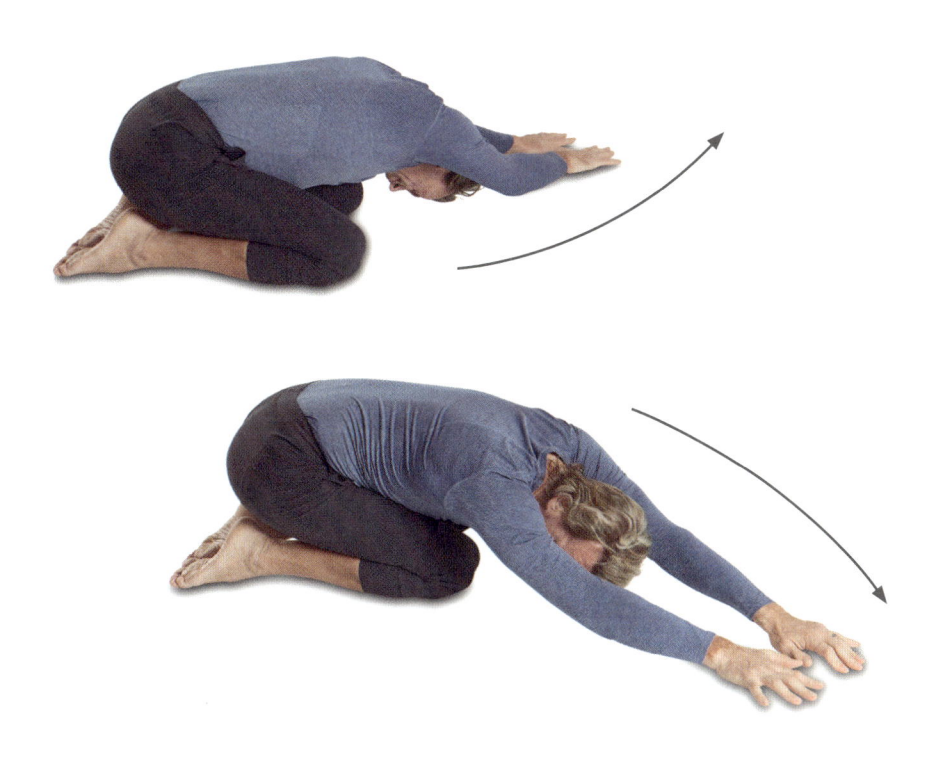

- From all fours, sit back on or close to your heels.
- Walk both hands around to the left.
- Spread your fingers and press both hands into the floor.
- Imagine they are stuck to the floor, then lean away from them to feel a deep side stretch.
- Walk both hands round to the right side and repeat.

REPS: Two on each side.

PLAY: Try stacking one hand on top of the other and briefly interlinking the fingers to anchor the hands to the floor.

MOVE 2: Cat Play

STEP 3

THUMBS UP

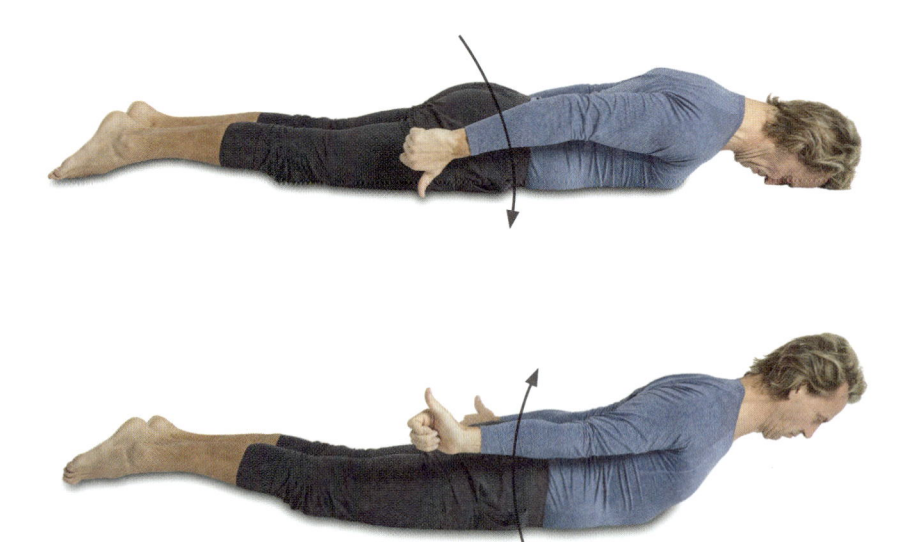

- Lie on your front with your arms close to your sides.
- Make a 'thumbs up' position with your hands but point the thumbs downwards.
- As you inhale, lift your whole body off the floor. Keep looking down.
- Point your thumbs up and squeeze your shoulder blades closer.
- As you exhale, lower your body back on to the floor.
- Continue to lift and lower.

REPS: Four.

STEP 4

COBRA FLOW

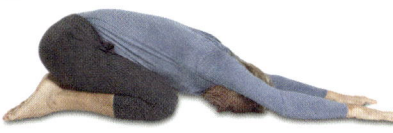

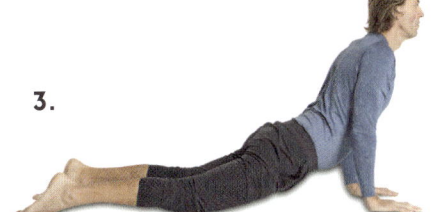

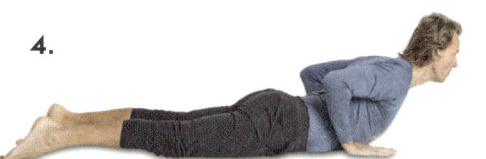

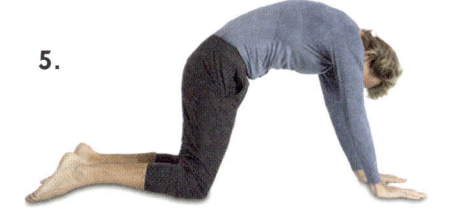

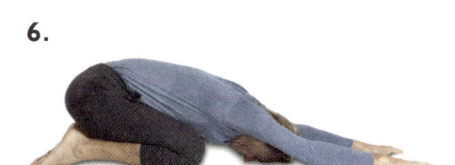

1.
2.
3.
4.
5.
6.

- Sit back on or close to your heels and stretch your arms overhead, palms down.
- As you inhale, rise up to Cat – all fours with a rounded back.
- As you exhale, drop your hips towards the floor and lower on to your front, keeping your hands under your shoulders.
- As you inhale, push into your hands and lift your upper body into Cobra (as far as is comfortable for the lower back).
- As you exhale, sit back on or close to your heels.
- Repeat.

REPS: Four.

MOVE 2: Cat Play

STEP 5

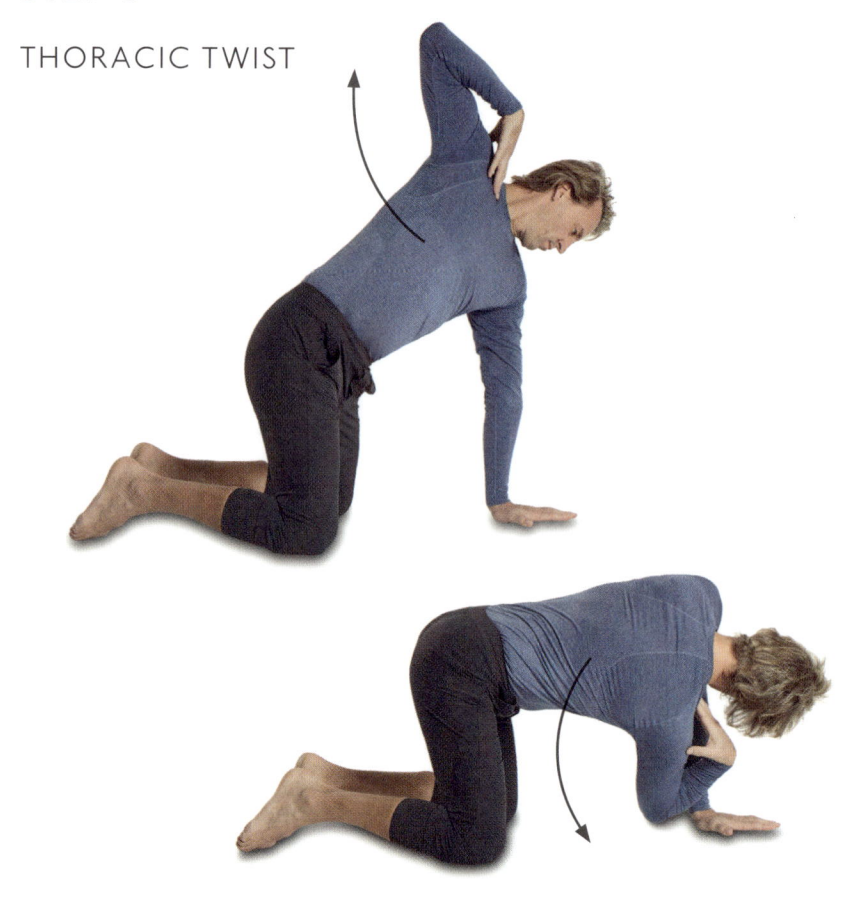

THORACIC TWIST

- Return to all fours but move your knees a little wider than hip-width apart.
- Place your right fingertips on your right shoulder.
- As you inhale, point your right elbow up to the ceiling without looking up.
- As you exhale, point your right elbow under your left armpit.
- Complete the reps and switch arms.

REPS: Five on each side.

PLAY: Try this technique with your right hand on your mid- or upper back, palm facing up. Lift and lower the shoulder five times.

STEP 6

FREESTYLE CAT

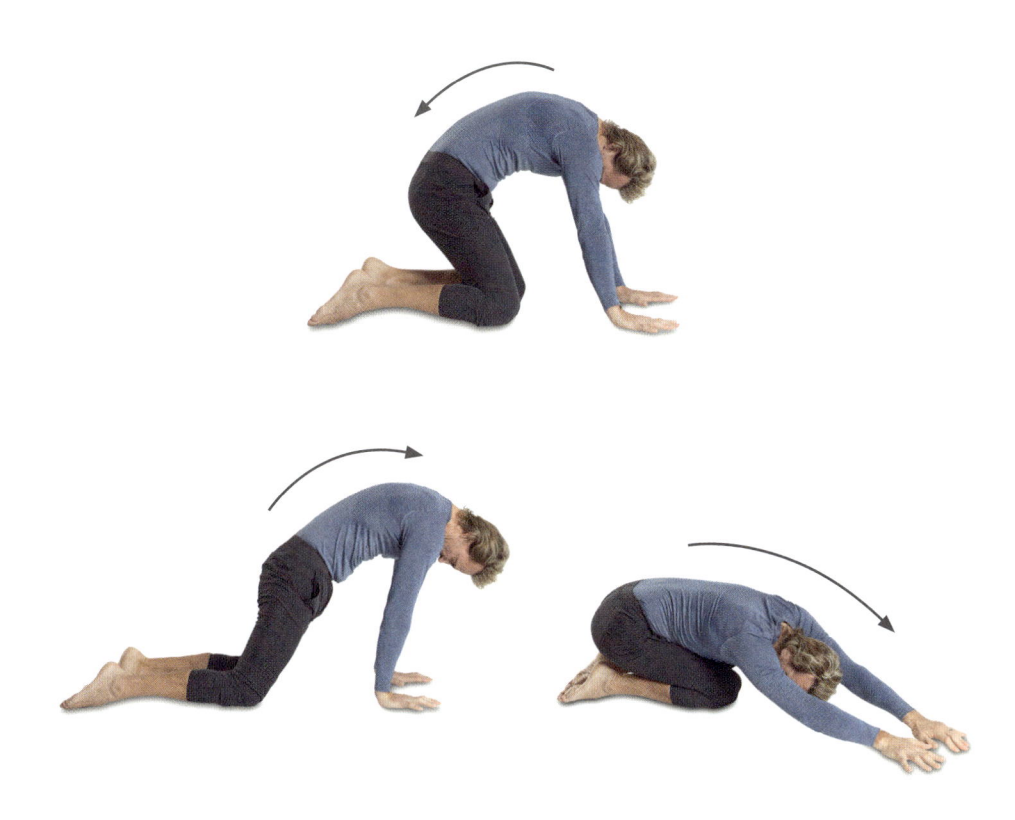

- Combine all the movements previously practised in this free-form flow.
- Start on all fours and close your eyes.
- Sit back on your heels, walk your hands to the side (Side Crawling), return to the start position, rise into Cobra and turn your head from side to side.
- Then just explore these movements in any order. Move in slow motion, breathing in and out through your nose. Try to work out where you feel tightest. Shoulders? Lower back? Neck?

REPS: Just flow and breathe.

PLAY: Invent your own exploratory movements that release your tightest spots.

MOVE 3
UNSTICK THE HIPS

'Sticky' or stiff hips can cause lower backache and curb your enjoyment of the sports you love. Here's a sequence to unlock the hips and glutes through circling, sweeping reps that gradually restore range of movement to create happy hips that move as they should.

This sequence is the solvent to unglue hips that feel stuck or stiff. It targets the outer hips, especially the backside or 'glutes' and iliotibial band, which runs down the outer thigh. We'll also loosen up those inner thigh and groin muscles with a few cross-legged flows and Butterfly Folds.

Like all the Moves, though, these techniques expand beyond the target anatomical area to stretch a host of other muscles that branch off the hips and could affect hip freedom of movement.

If your hips feel really 'sticky' this routine would pair perfectly with the next Move, Lunge Flow, which focuses on the hip flexors, located at the front of the hips. Together, the two Moves tick all the hip mobility boxes.

You may have spotted that there are some cross-legged techniques. I appreciate that many adults may not have sat cross-legged since they were at junior school, and for some it is impossible or uncomfortable. Men particularly can struggle with the position, partly due to the narrower shape of the male pelvis. If your knees are too high or it strains your back, either try sitting with the soles of the feet together or turn to the Gentle version of Unstick the Hips.

If tight buttocks or 'glutes' are an issue (which can literally manifest as a pain in the backside!) you have come to the right place. Steps 4–6 are fantastic for loosening those muscles but also try the technique suggested in Play at the end of 90/90 Drops and hold it for a good 20 seconds or more. This stretch can get pretty intense so don't forget to smile and breathe. The promise of supple hips awaits.

STEP 1

HIP CIRCLING

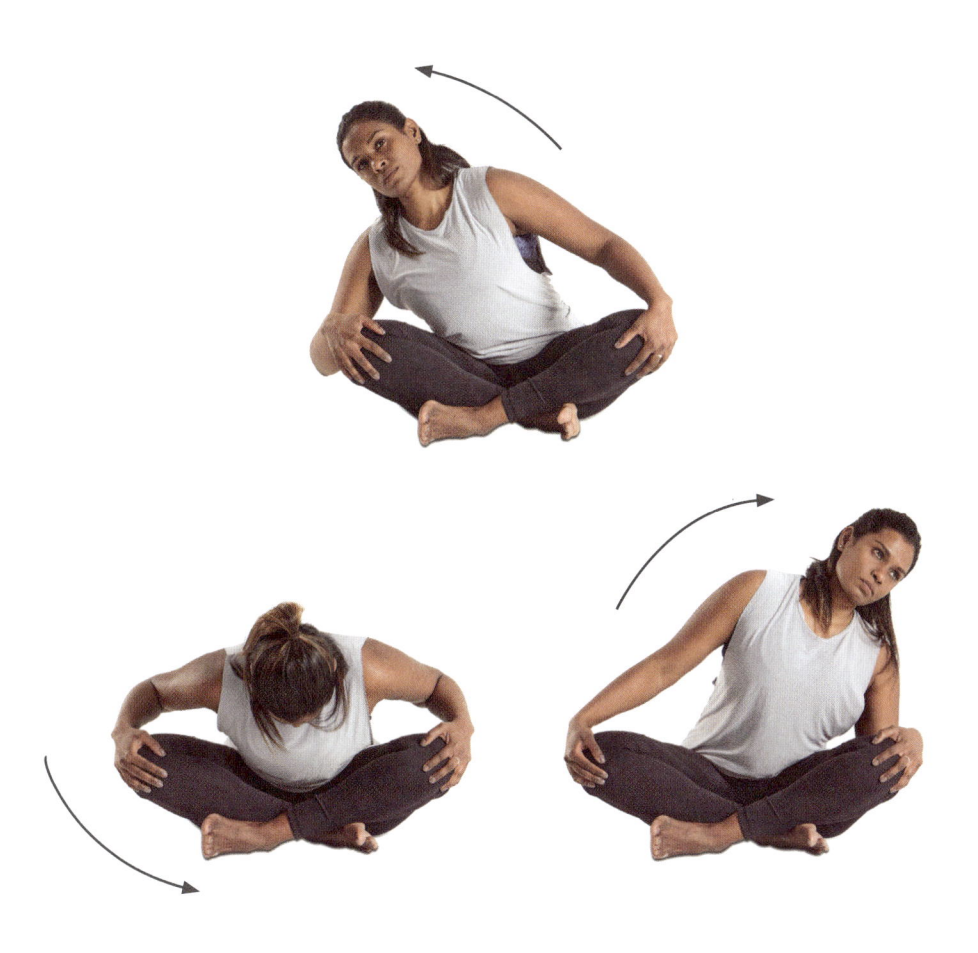

- Sit cross-legged, or with the soles of the feet together.
- Place your hands on your knees.
- Slowly swing your upper body around in circles.
- Breathe in and out as you circle.

REPS: Six.

MOVE 3: Unstick the Hips

STEP 2

SIDE SWEEPS

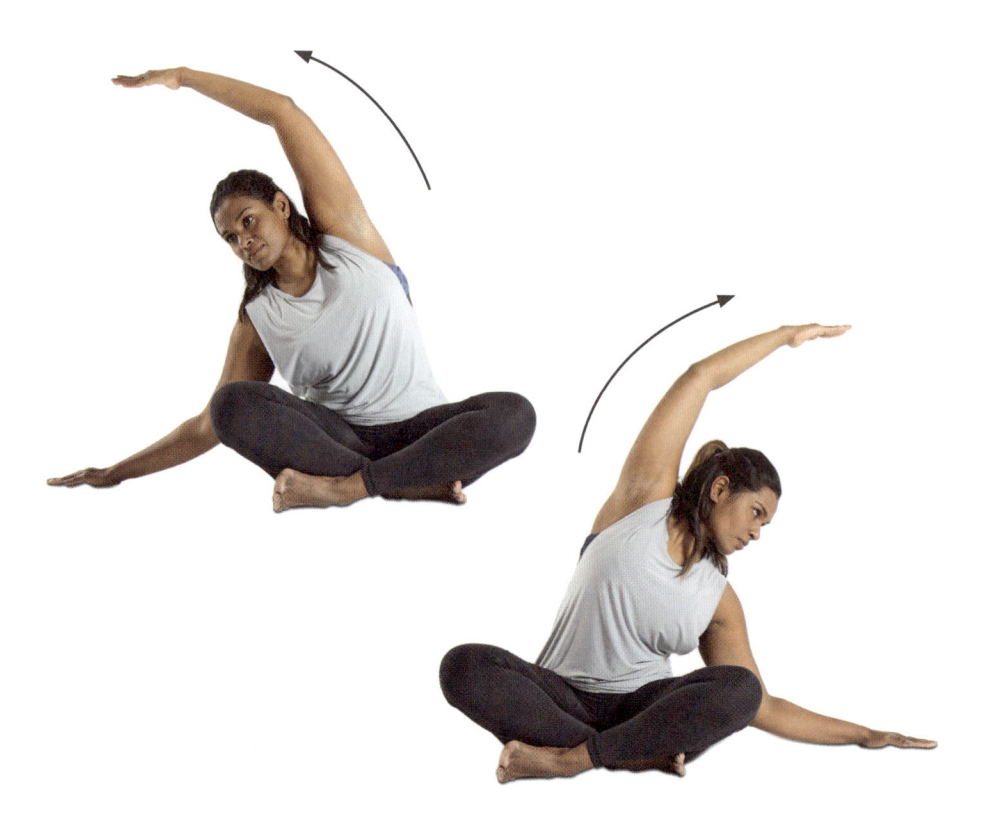

- Stay cross-legged and sit tall.
- Place your fingertips on the floor on either side of your body.
- Exhale, reach your right arm up and lean to the left side, sweeping the arm over.
- Inhale and return to the centre.
- Exhale, reach your left arm up and lean to the right, sweeping the arm over.
- Continue to flow from side to side, inhaling into the centre and exhaling to the side.

REPS: Four–six on each side.

TIP: Close your eyes in Side Sweeps for better body awareness. Is one side tighter than the other?

STEP 3

BUTTERFLY FOLDS

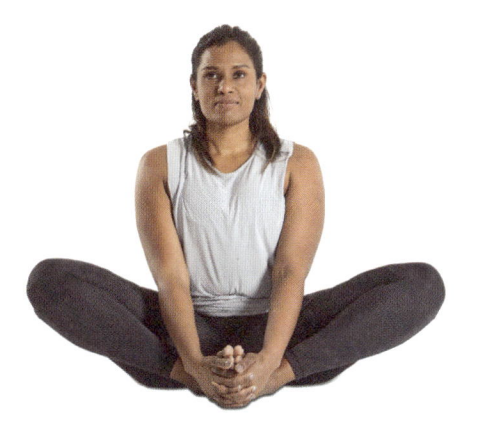

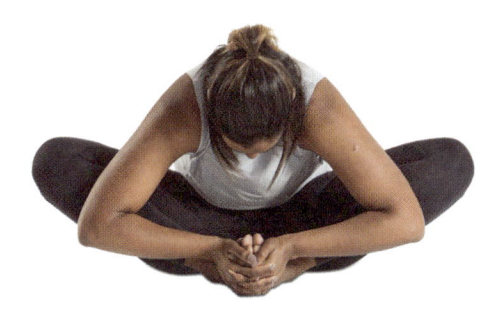

- Place the soles of your feet together and let the knees drop out.
- Either wrap your hands around your feet or hold on to your ankles.
- As you inhale, sit tall by lengthening your spine and lifting your chest.
- As you exhale, flex your back and fold forwards, bringing your head towards your feet.
- Continue lifting and folding.

REPS: Five.

MOVE 3: Unstick the Hips

STEP 4

90/90 DROPS

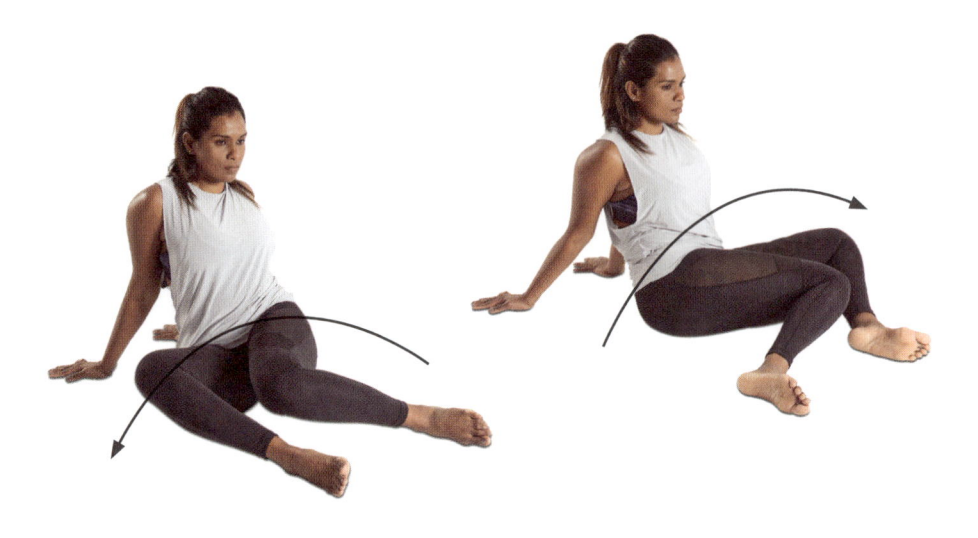

- Sit tall with your legs bent into a 90-degree position and your feet flat on the floor, a little wider than hip-width apart.
- Lean back, rest your hands on the floor and lift your chest.
- Keeping your feet stuck to the floor, drop both knees to the right, then the left, swaying them from side to side. Roll on to the edges of your feet.
- Breathe in and out as you sway the legs.

REPS: Six–eight.

PLAY: Return to the start position. Place your right ankle on top of your left thigh and lift the chest. Slowly sway your legs from side to side. Repeat on the other side.

MOVE

STEP 5

90 DROP AND TWIST

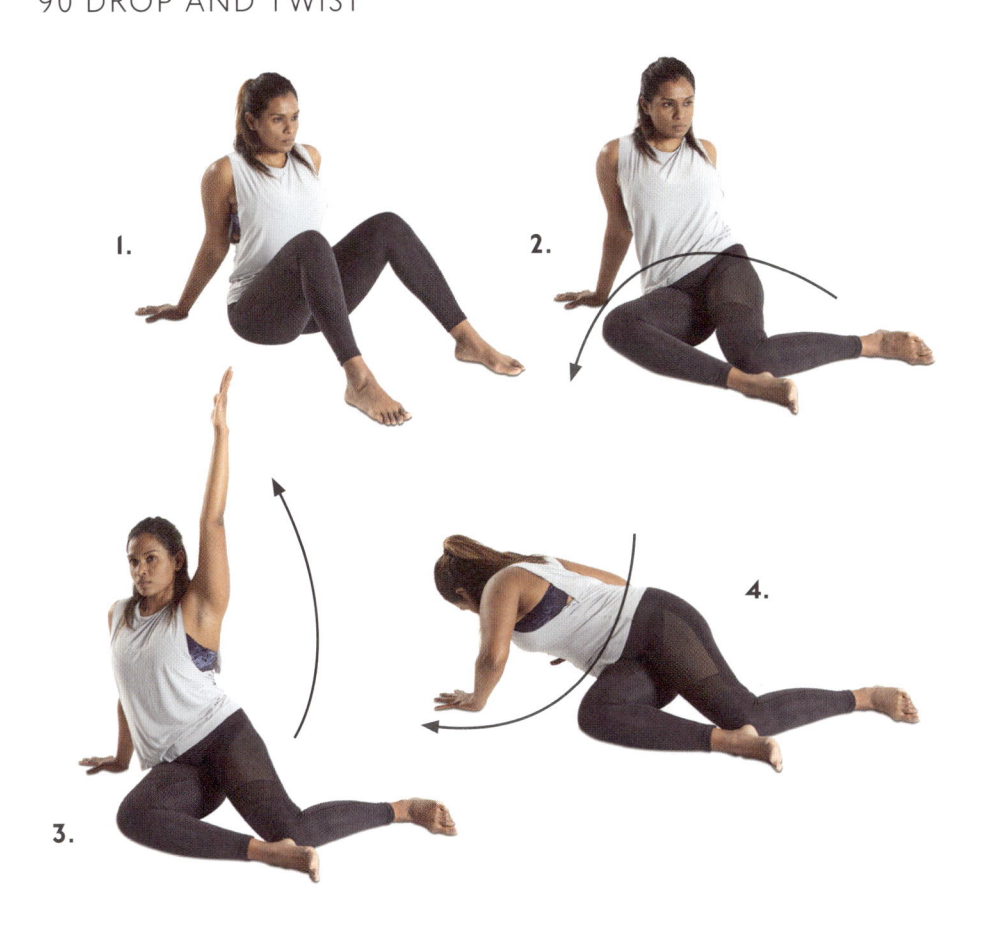

- Adopt the 90/90 Drops start position.
- Perform a 90/90 Drop to the right by lowering your knees to the floor.
- Lift your left hand off the floor and rotate your torso to the right.
- Sweep your left hand round and place it close to your right hand. Bend your arms a little and drop your chest towards the floor.
- Return to the start position and repeat on the other side.

REPS: Three on each side.

MOVE 3: Unstick the Hips

STEP 6

HUG AND TWIST

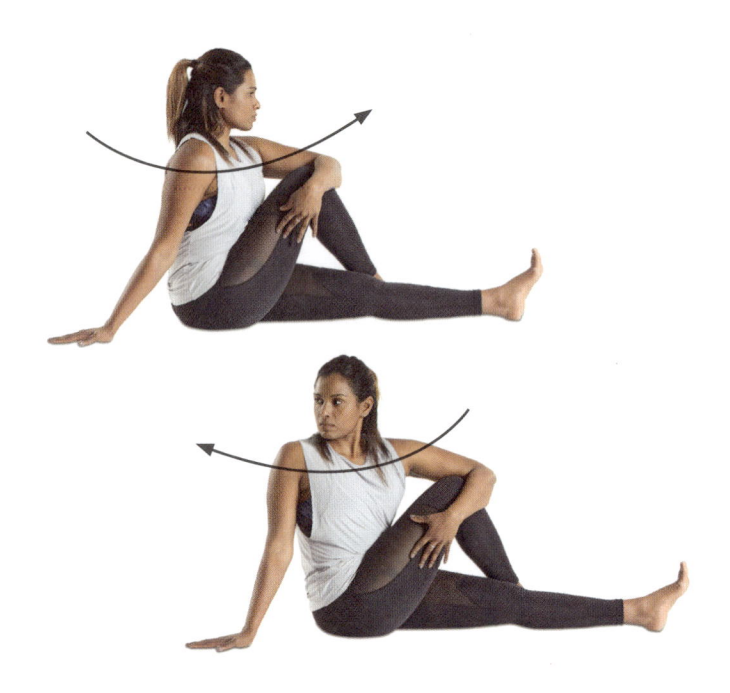

- Straighten out your left leg.
- Step your right foot over your left thigh.
- Wrap your left arm around your right leg and hug it towards you.
- Place your right hand behind your back.
- Exhale and turn your shoulders to the right.
- Inhale and turn your shoulders to face the front.
- Repeat by gently twisting the upper body to the right and back.
- Unravel the legs and repeat on the other side.

REPS: Four on each side.

CHANGE IT UP

If you want it tougher...
Try the Advanced version of this Move on page 146.

If you want it more gentle...
For a less-strenuous version of this Move, see page 100.

MOVE

MOVE 4
LUNGE FLOW

Do you spend hours each day hunched over a computer? Your body is crying out to flip that slouch into reverse, and a lunge is just the tonic. By lengthening the spine, rolling back those shoulders and 'opening' the hips a lunge offers much-needed medicine for modern working life, and an end to lower backache. You could even say 'a lunge a day keeps the physio away'.

Why do lunges get their own sequence? The life-enhancing, posture-improving lunge is an antidote to the slouch, really 'opening' up the whole of the front of the body, which feels fantastic if you spend eight hours a day folded over a laptop.

Picture your typical seated stance either at work or driving: flexed shoulders spine and hips. Now flip that posture into reverse by drawing the shoulders back, puffing out the chest and stepping a leg back to stretch the front of the hip. Result? The extension your body is craving.

In terms of hip and leg muscles, lunges target the upper quads and the hip flexors – the iliopsoas muscles, located where the front of the thigh meets the hip. Anyone who does a sport that requires repetitive leg lifting, such as hiking, running or cycling, will be well aware of how tight hip flexors feel. But people who sit a lot are also advised to stretch these muscles because tight hip flexors are a big contributor to lower backache.

The lunge is held throughout the sequence to ensure the hip flexors get a good long stretch while we distract ourselves playing with upper body movements.

If you find kneeling uncomfortable place a foam yoga/Pilates block under your back knee or grab a cushion from the sofa. Alternatively, try the Gentle version of Lunge Flow, which is done with the back knee lifted off the floor.

> **Start with your right leg forwards and move through the entire flow, then repeat the sequence with the left foot in front.**

STEP 1

SLIDING

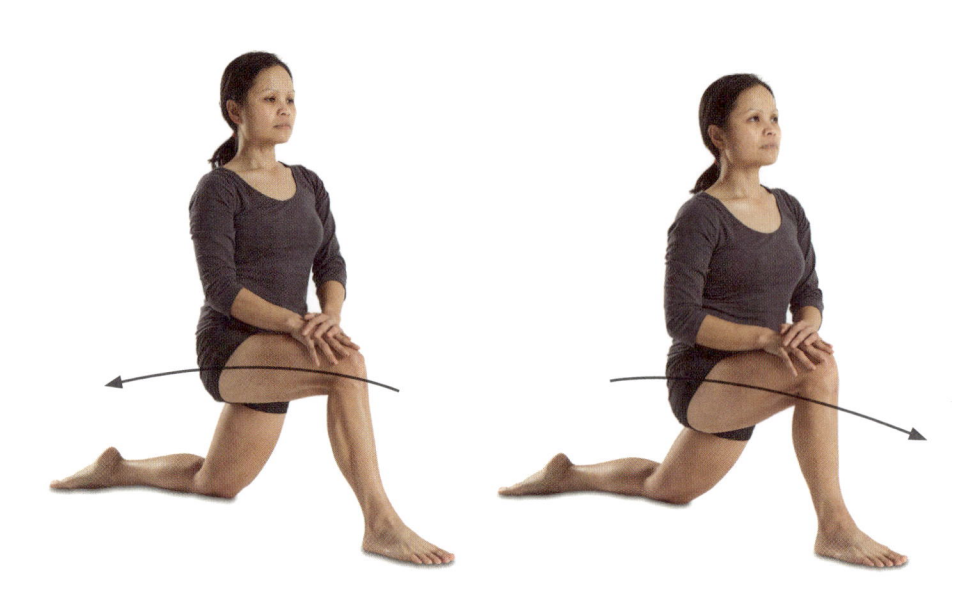

- Start on all fours.
- Step your right foot up in between your hands.
- Lift your upper body and place both hands on your front thigh.
- Lean slightly back and tuck in your backside. Inhale here.
- As you exhale, slide forwards and sink into the lunge, keeping your backside tucked in.
- Inhale to slide back up, then repeat.
- Continue sliding back and forth.

REPS: Four

STEP 2

ELBOW CIRCLING

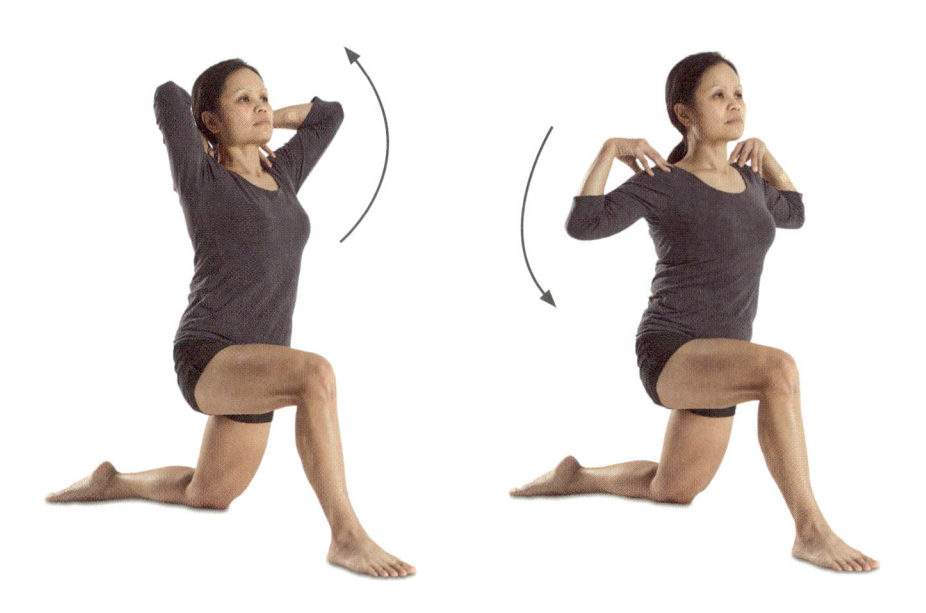

- Place both hands lightly on top of your shoulders.
- Make slow circles with both elbows.

REPS: Six (three forwards and three backwards).

PLAY: Switch to a swimming motion by circling alternate elbows forwards or backwards.

MOVE 4: Lunge Flow

STEP 3

ELBOW TWISTING

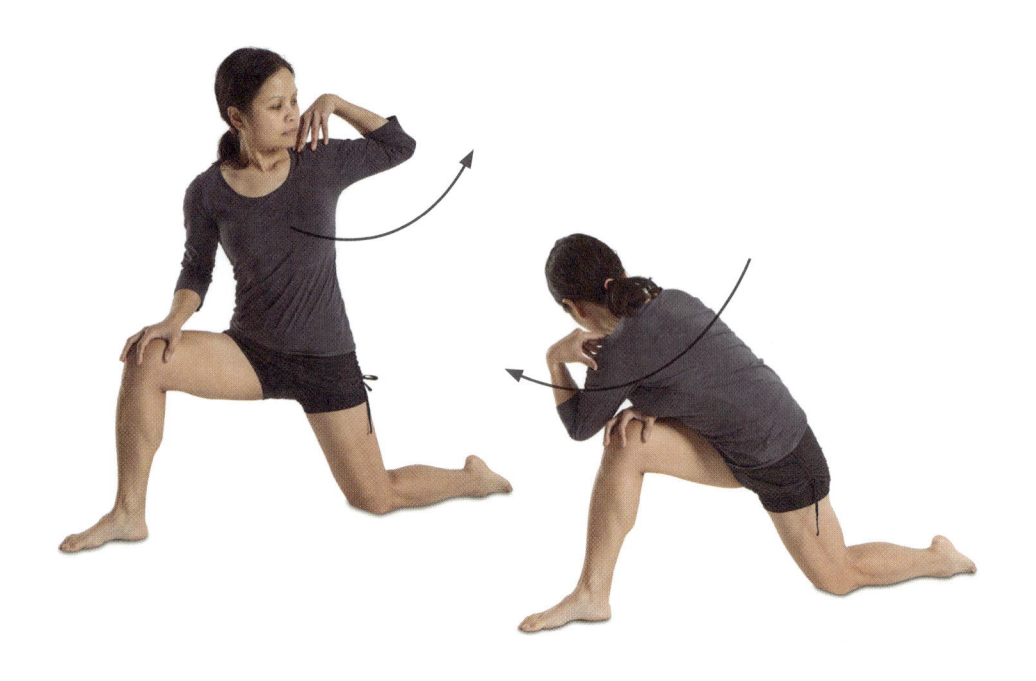

- From Elbow Circling, keep your left hand on your left shoulder. Drop your right hand to rest on your right thigh.
- As you inhale, point your left elbow behind you.
- As you exhale, sweep your left elbow across your body and point it down to the floor.
- Continue, pointing the elbow back and down for the specified number of reps,.

REPS: Four

MOVE

STEP 4

LUNGE WAVING

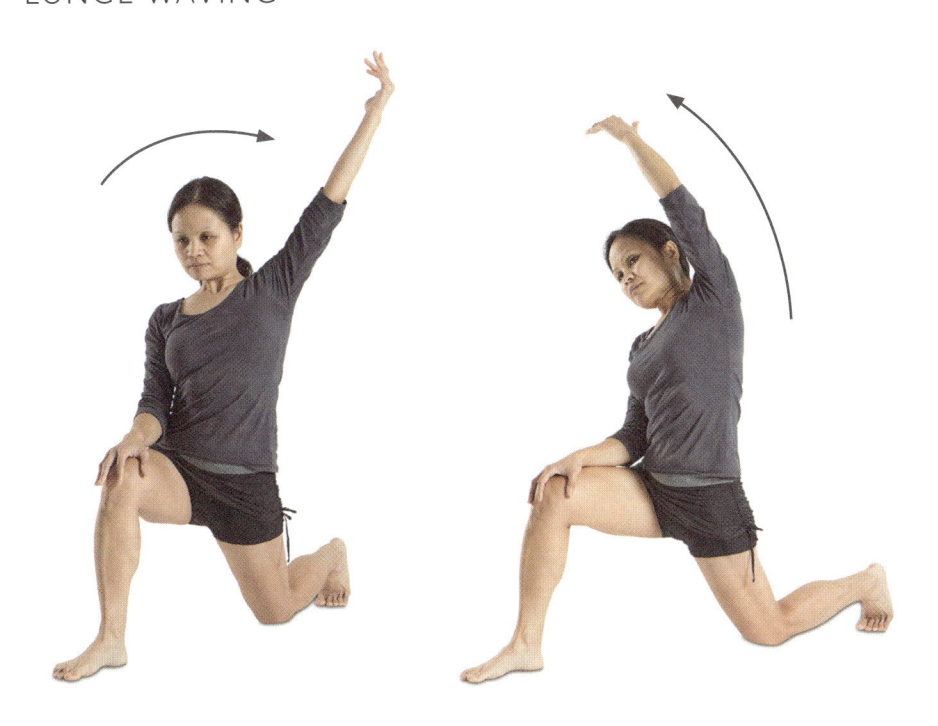

- Reach your left arm up above your head. Keep your right hand on your thigh. Inhale here.
- As you exhale, sweep your left arm over to your right side.
- Repeat, inhaling to the centre and exhaling over for the specified number of reps.

REPS: Four

PLAY: Try sweeping the arm across the body to create more of a twist.

MOVE 4: Lunge Flow

STEP 5

LUNGE TWISTING

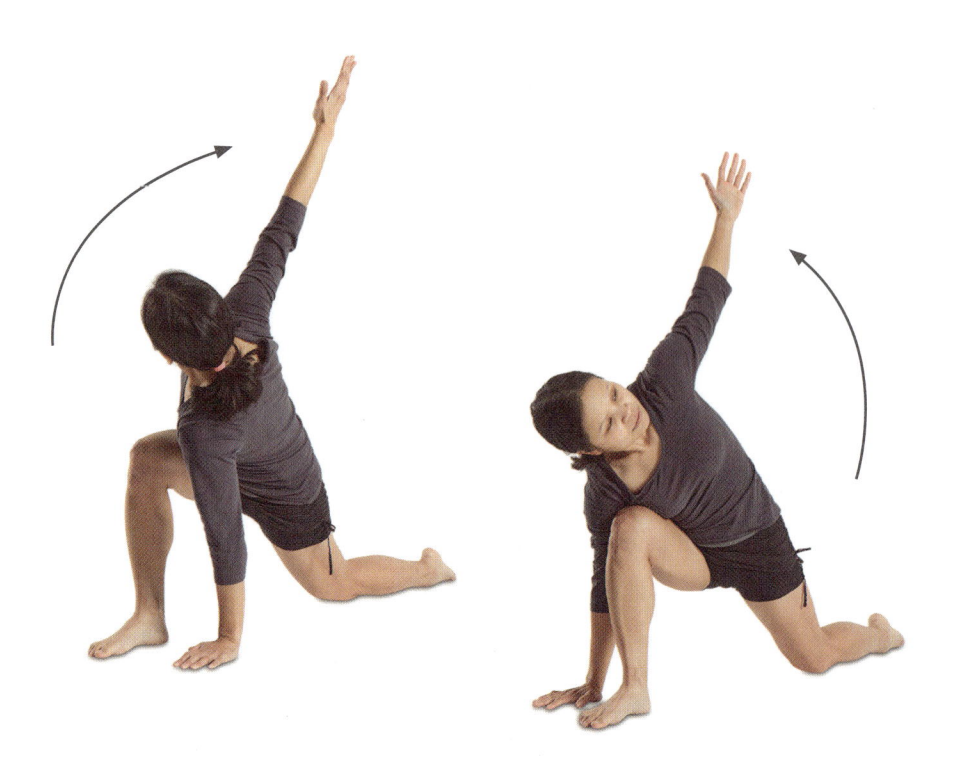

- Drop both hands to the floor on either side of your front foot.
- As you inhale, reach your right arm up.
- As you exhale, return it to the floor.
- As you inhale, reach your left arm up.
- As you exhale, return it to the floor.
- Continue to twist side to side for the specified number of reps.

REPS: Six

60 MOVE

STEP 6

SIDE LUNGING

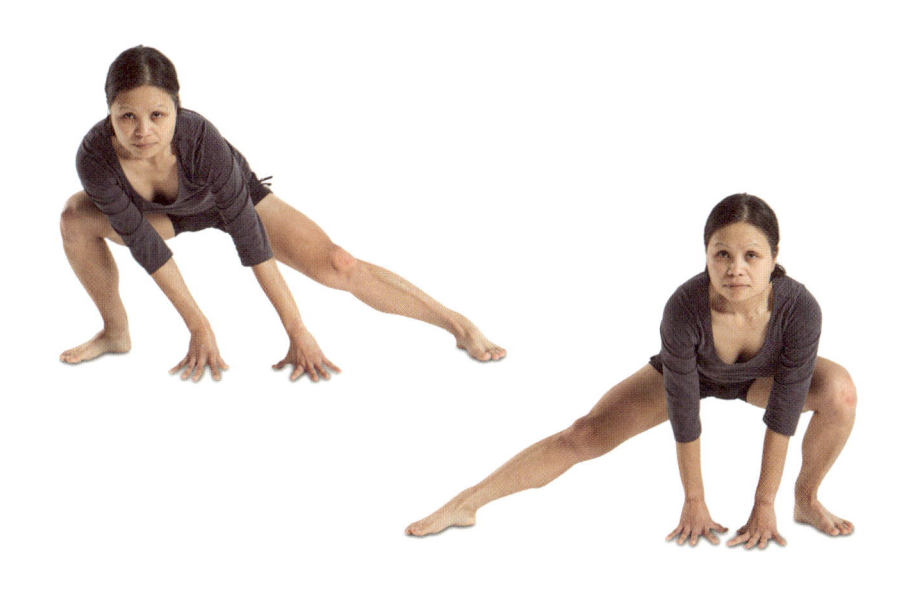

- Move your feet wider apart and turn your toes slightly outwards.
- Place your fingertips on the floor.
- Crawl your hands towards your right foot, bending your right leg and straightening your left.
- Crawl your hands back to the centre.
- Crawl your hands over to your left foot, bending your left leg and straightening your right.
- Check that the bending knee tracks in line with your big toe as you lunge.
- Keep your breathing steady and slow.

REPS: Four

MOVE 4: Lunge Flow

MOVE 5
HAMSTRING RELEASING

If locked hamstrings are wreaking havoc with your running, football or cycling then they may need a little liberating. This is an energetic, active solution that should satisfy even the more stretch-averse athlete. We're not talking about doing the splits or even touching our toes, just working to make muscles less injury-prone so they will let you run, kick or pedal to your heart's content.

Can't touch your toes? You are by no means alone. Many of us lose this ability to reach the ground somewhere around puberty, but we can regain a little of this long-lost hamstring flexibility by playing with these swinging, rocking and swaying movements.

This routine would suit a range of sports lovers, from soccer fans to runners or tennis players, especially as some of the movements mimic the running stance. It would make a useful warm-up sequence for any of these sports, but would also suit those who have a sedentary job whereby these muscles rarely get lengthened, often contributing to lower back niggles.

Hamstrings are sensitive to being stretched too hard and fast so go in softly and never feel you must lock the leg straight. Think about coming to the 'edge' of the stretch and then ease out again as you perform your reps, and keep a slow, deep breathing rhythm.

Of course, our hamstrings don't exist in isolation so this Move extends down to the calves and up into the hips and lower back.

If your hamstrings are particularly tight, end the sequence by returning to Swaying (step 4) but just hang out here for a good 30 seconds, relaxing the upper body.

Please note: If you have very tight hamstrings or any lower back issues, turn to the Gentle version of Hamstring Releasing on page 108. It is probably a better place to start building flexibility and is super-gentle on the lower back.

As always, feel free to play with the movements where you see the Play sign, and even when you don't.

STEP 1

RELAXED LEG SWINGS

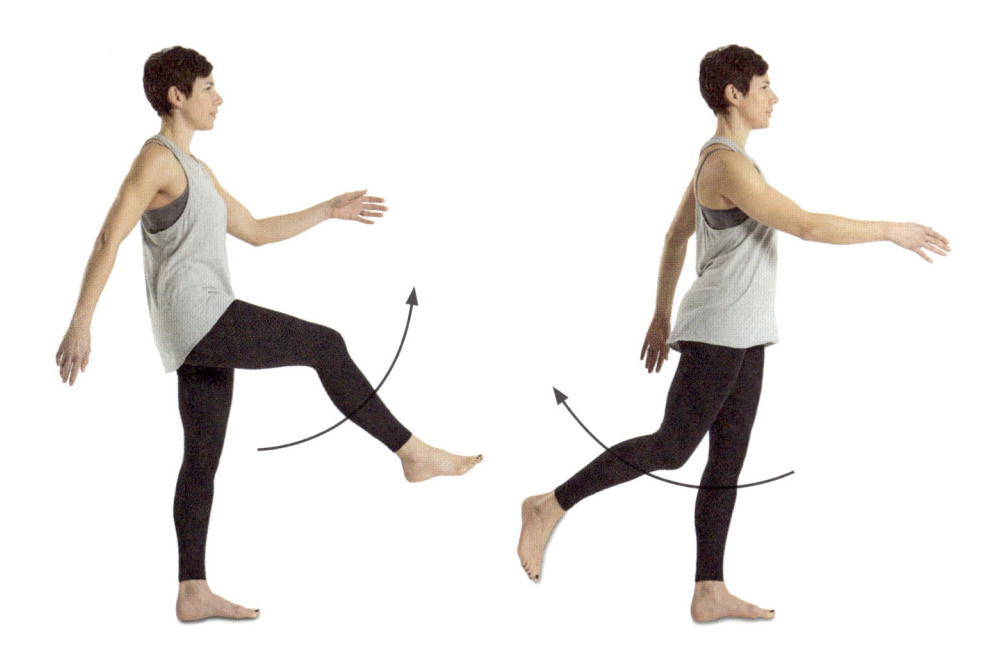

- Stand tall with your arms relaxed by your sides.
- Shift your weight on to your left leg.
- Lift your right foot just off the floor and start swinging the leg back and forth. Keep your swinging leg a little bent. Bend your arms, too, and swing them the opposite way, as if you are running.
- Lift the swinging leg just high enough to feel a slight hamstring stretch at the back of the thigh.
- Move slowly and smoothly, breathing through the nose.
- Complete the reps, then switch legs.

REPS: Six–eight on each side.

STEP 2
STRAIGHT LEG SWINGS

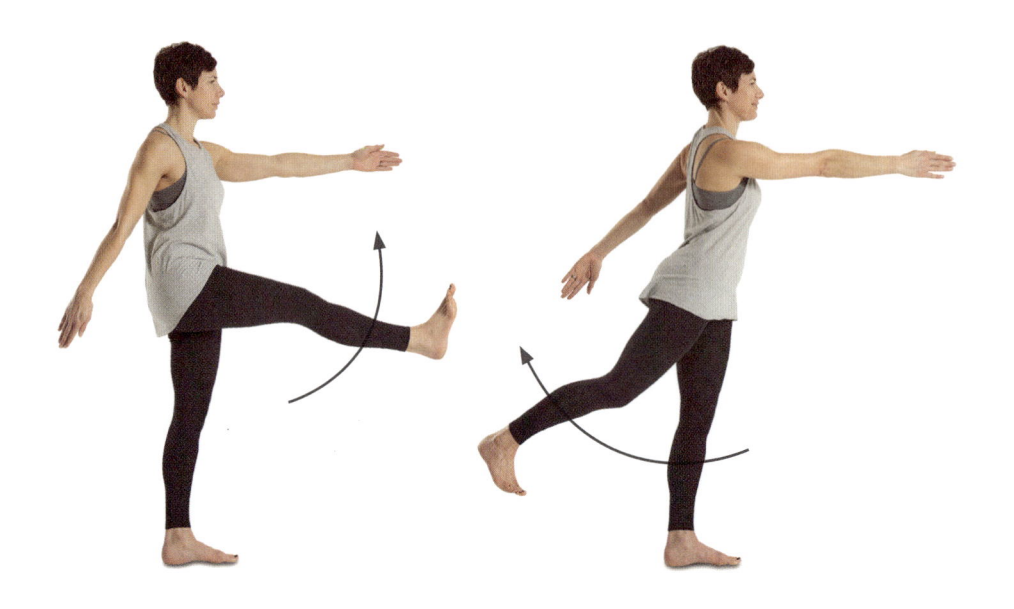

- Shift your weight back on to your left leg.
- Stretch your arms out to the sides, to shoulder height.
- Swing your right leg up and back but keep it straight.
- Gradually increase the height of the leg on each swing, but avoid stretching the hamstrings too deeply too soon.
- Move slowly and smoothly, breathing through the nose.
- Complete the reps, then switch legs.

REPS: Six–eight on each side.

STEP 3

FORWARD TIPS

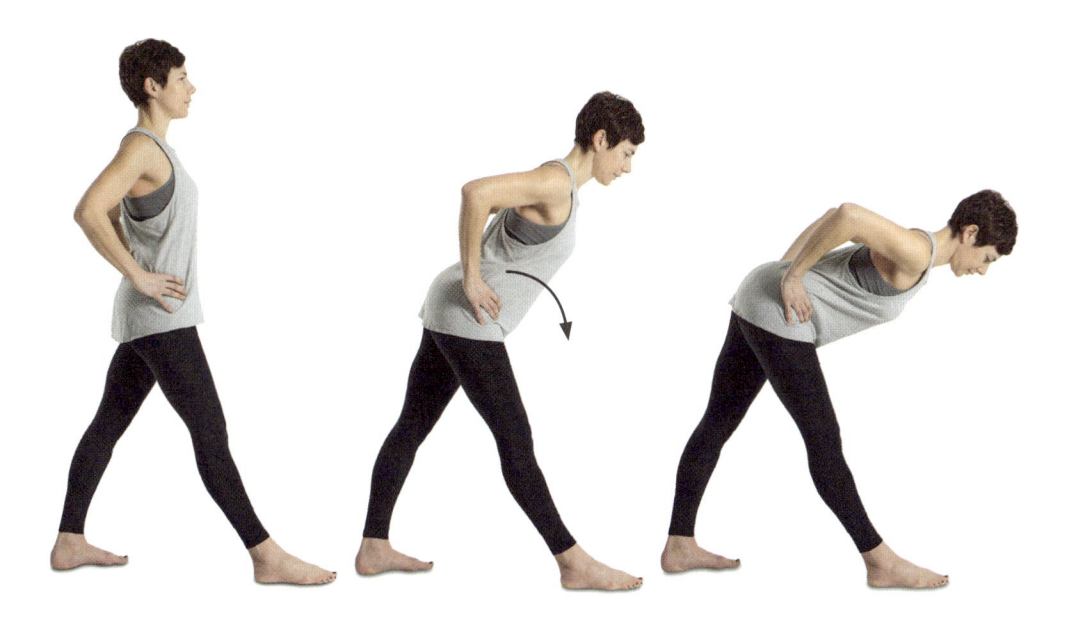

- Stand with your hands on your hips and your feet hip-width apart.
- Take a step forwards with your right leg. Keep your feet parallel and both legs straight.
- Exhale and tip your upper body forwards, keeping your back straight, until you feel a gentle hamstring stretch.
- To exit, inhale, engage the core and rise back up.
- Complete the reps, then switch legs.

REPS: Six on each side.

MOVE 5: Hamstring Releasing

STEP 4

SWAYING

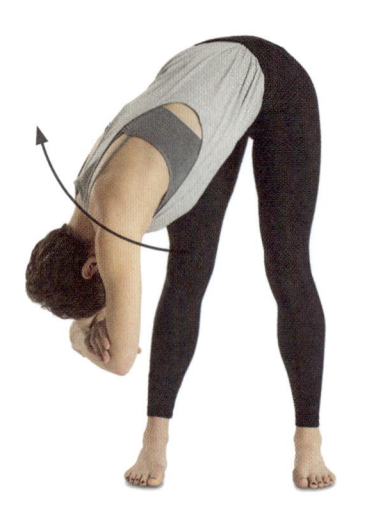

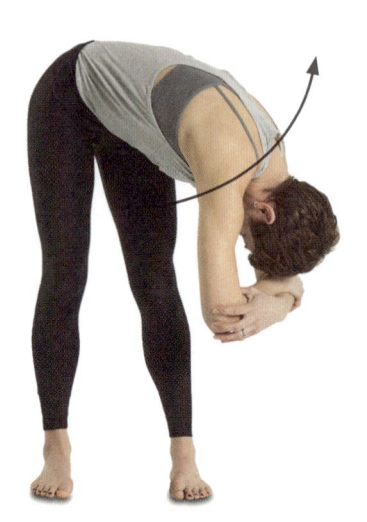

- Stand with your feet hip-width apart.
- Exhale, bend your knees, relax your arms and roll down into a forward bend slowly and gradually, by tucking in your chin and allowing the spine to flex.
- Fold your arms and relax your head completely.
- Sway slowly from side to side, breathing through the nose.
- To return to standing, bend your knees, relax your arms and roll slowly back up to standing.

REPS: Just roll down once and sway for 10–15 seconds or longer.

TIP: Bend the knees slightly if the hamstrings feel tight.

STEP 5

WALKING DOG

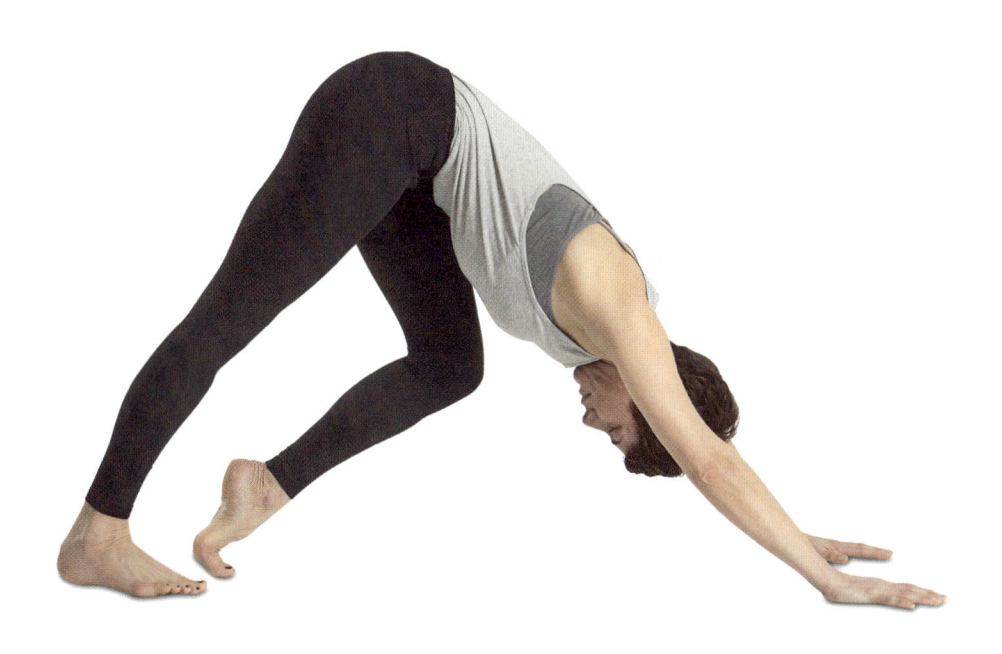

- From the Swaying position, bend your knees and drop your hands to the floor.
- Walk your hands forwards until your body forms a triangle position, or Downward Dog, with your feet hip-width apart.
- 'Walk' the dog by bending one leg and pushing the other heel down.
- Continue to walk on the spot from leg to leg, breathing in and out as you move.

REPS: Walk for 10 seconds or longer.

MOVE 5: Hamstring Releasing

STEP 6

ROCK THE HAMMIES

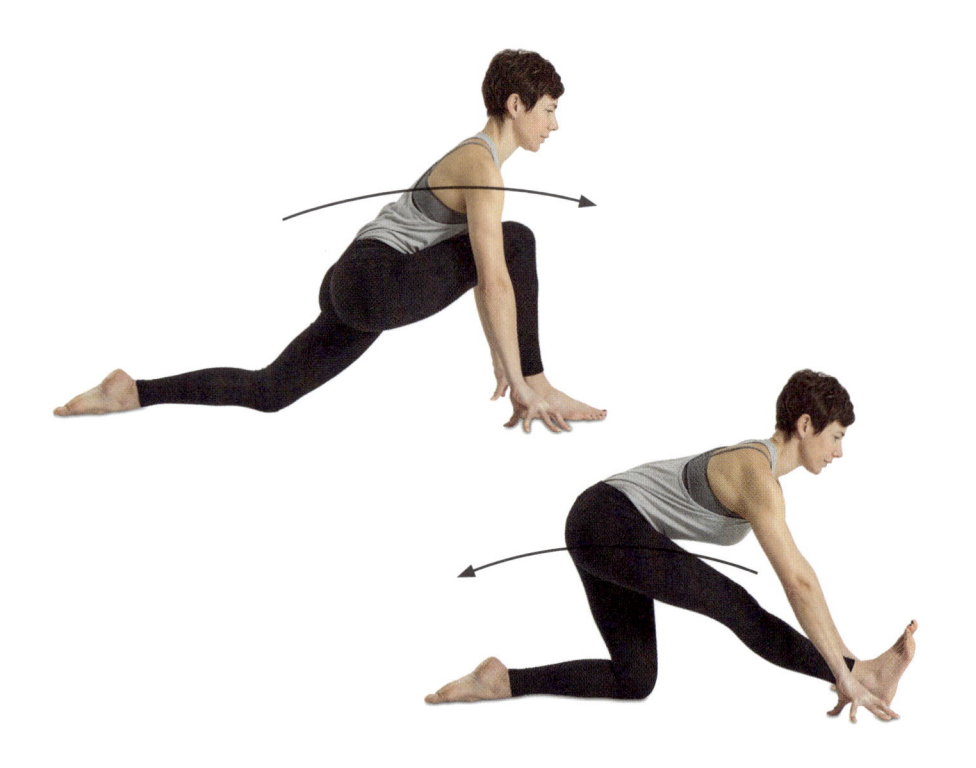

- From Walking Dog, lower your left knee to the floor (padding it with a cushion if required) and step your right foot up between your hands.
- Bend your right leg, positioning the knee above the ankle. Place your fingertips either side of your front foot in a sprint start position.
- As you inhale, drop your hips and sink lower into the lunge.
- As you exhale, move your hips back, straighten your right leg a little and roll on to your right heel, toes pointing up.
- Repeat, rocking forwards and backwards to complete the reps, then switch legs.

REPS: Six on each side.

PLAY: Try a few rocks keeping the sole of the front foot on the floor.

MOVE

MOVE 6
SHOULDER FLOSSING

Unshackle your shoulders! This sequence uses smooth, gliding, 'flossing' movement to release tight muscles and tease out knots – the 'motion is lotion' principle. Goodbye 'sore and achy', hello 'light and tingly'. This repetitive sliding action, done with a strap or tie, also works to gradually restore the flexibility of this naturally highly mobile joint.

This sequence can serve purely to warm up the shoulders for sport or be used as a therapeutic aid to systematically release upper body tension.

Our shoulders, which comprise a shallow ball-and-socket joint, are designed to be the most flexible joint in the body. They let us scratch an itch in the middle of our backs, perform a tennis serve, do the butterfly stroke, strike a golf ball, and a whole host of other complicated movements. However, shoulders are also prone to tension and tightness around the anterior shoulder and chest muscles ('pecs') and this can contribute to a poor posture, through rounded shoulders.

This sequence is designed to target these postural muscles but goes on to ease out the surrounding shoulder muscle groups, resulting in improved overall shoulder flexibility.

You will need a cotton yoga strap, but a dressing gown belt or tie would work well. It's super easy to cheat and hunch your shoulders during these techniques so get your technique perfected early by trying this test:

'Stand tall' with your feet hip-distance apart and the core lightly engaged.

Raise the strap up, but keep your shoulders down. If this proves tricky, ask someone to stand behind you and place their hands on your shoulders until you've retrained the mind to kick this shoulder – hunching habit.

STEP 1

SHOULDER FLEXION

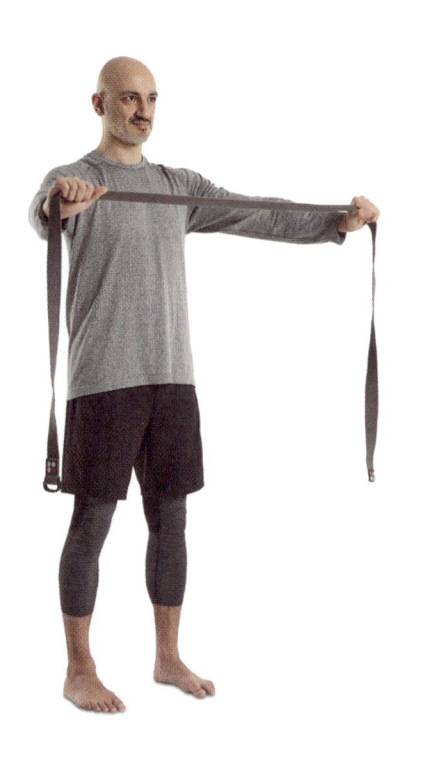

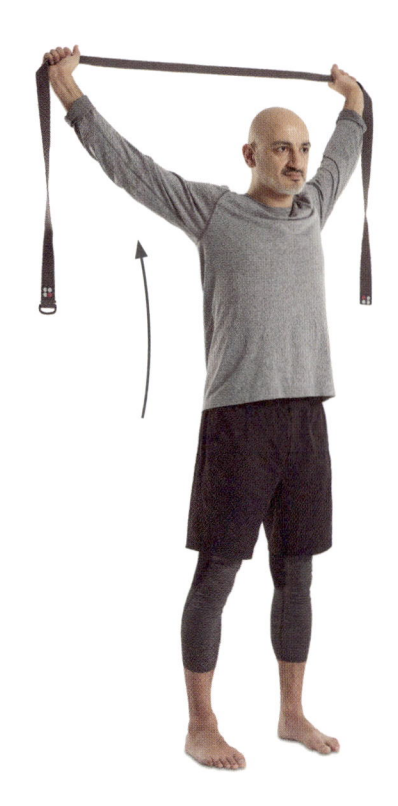

- Stand tall with your feet hip-width apart.
- Hold the strap in front of your body at chest height.
- Position your hands at least body-width apart, or wider, depending on the flexibility of your shoulders.
- As you inhale, raise your arms up above your head without lifting your shoulders.
- As you exhale, return your strap to chest height.
- Repeat, moving slowly and smoothly.

REPS: Five.

TIP: Practise raising your arms without lifting or hunching your shoulders.

STEP 2

SHOULDER EXTENSION

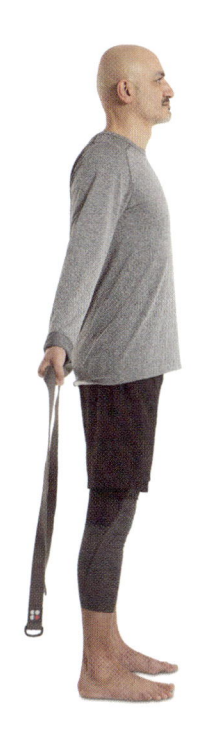

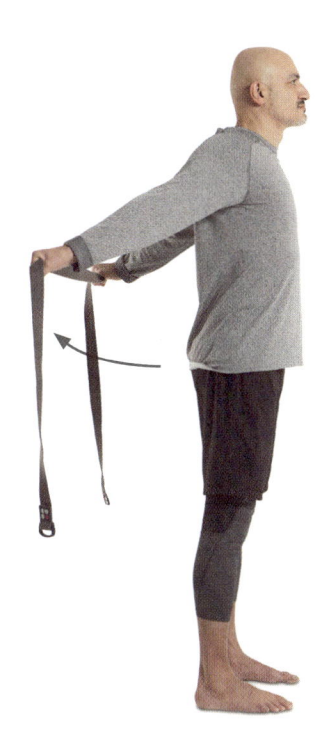

- Take the strap behind your back.
- Place your hands body-width apart with the palms facing forwards.
- As you inhale, raise the strap up behind you. Keep your arms straight and avoid leaning forwards.
- As you exhale, return the strap to the start position.
- Repeat. If the movement is limited, take the hands wider. If the movement is easy, position them closer together.

REPS: Five.

MOVE 6: Shoulder Flossing

STEP 3

BACK SCRATCHING

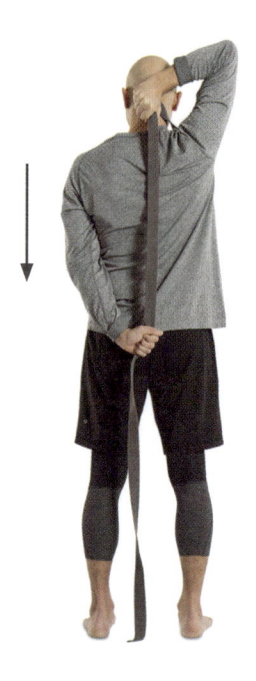

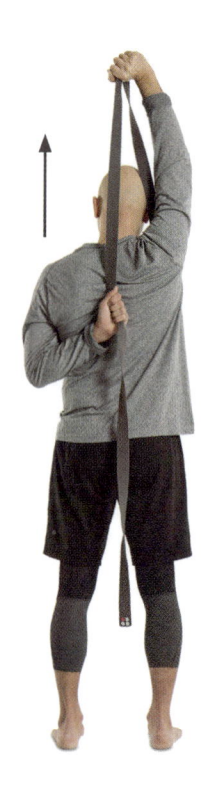

- Hold the strap above your head, as in Shoulder Flexion.
- Bend your right arm and drop your right hand behind your neck.
- Let go with the left hand so the strap drops free.
- Hold on to it again but grasp it much lower down.
- As you inhale, straighten the top arm so that it drags the bottom arm up your back.
- As you exhale, return the arms to the start point.
- Continue, sliding smoothly up and down. If movement is limited, take the hands further apart. If the movement is easy, position them closer together.
- Complete the reps, then switch arms.

REPS: Four–six on each side.

STEP 4

ELBOW CIRCLES

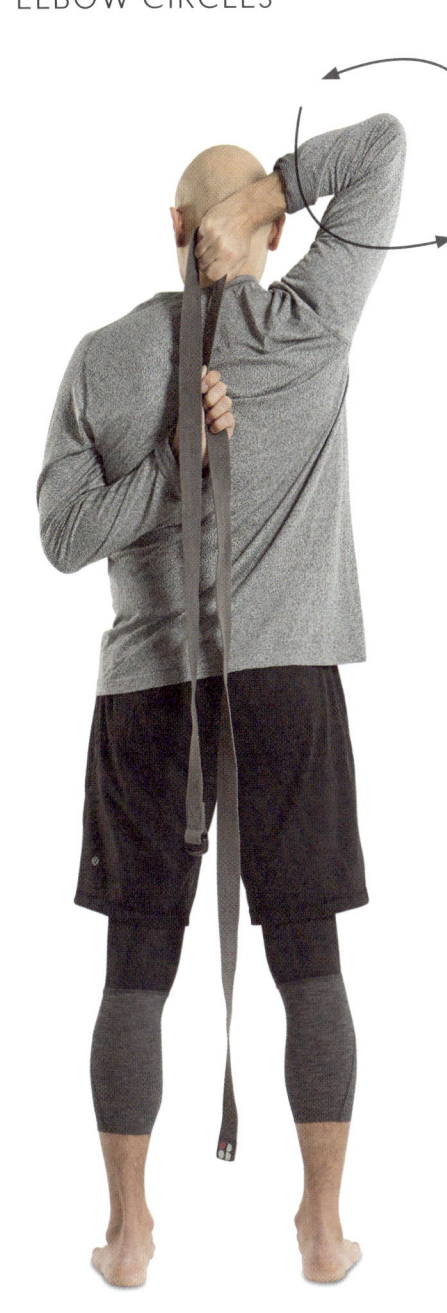

- Return your arms to the Back Scratching start position with the right arm holding the strap straight above your head and the left hand holding the strap lower down.
- Walk your hands closer together.
- Rotate the top elbow as if drawing small circles above your head.
- Breathe slowly through the nose.
- Complete the reps, then switch arms.

REPS: 10 (five clockwise and five anticlockwise).

MOVE 6: Shoulder Flossing

STEP 5

SIDE STRETCH

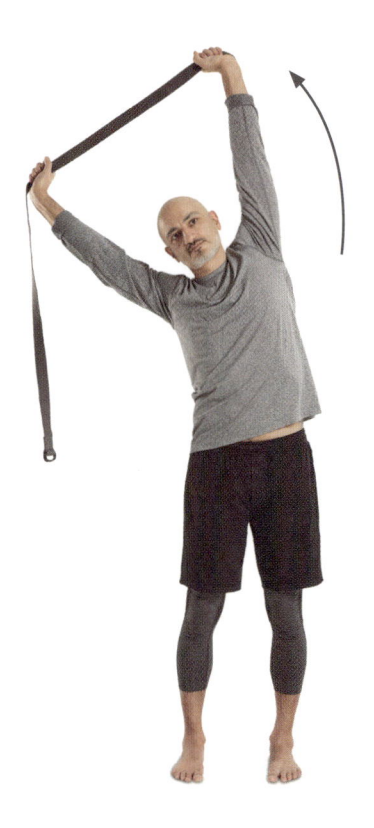

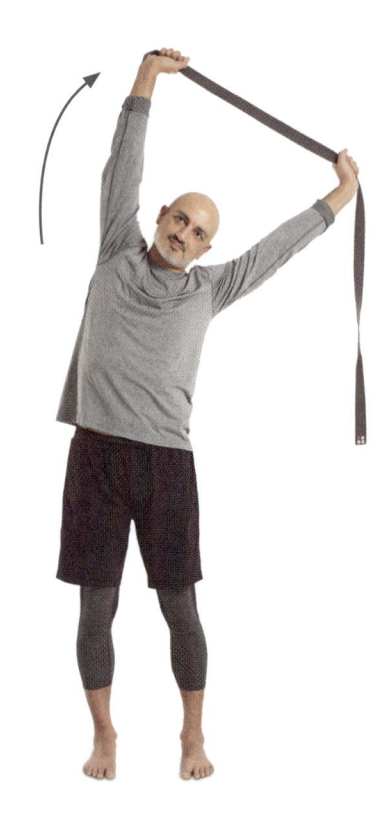

- Hold the strap above your head, as in Shoulder Flexion, but move your hands a little wider apart.
- Lean to the right side as you exhale, and sway your arms to the right.
- Inhale as you move back to the centre.
- Lean to the left side as you exhale, and sway your arms to the left.
- Continue to complete the reps.

REPS: Three on each side.

STEP 6

SIDE SWING

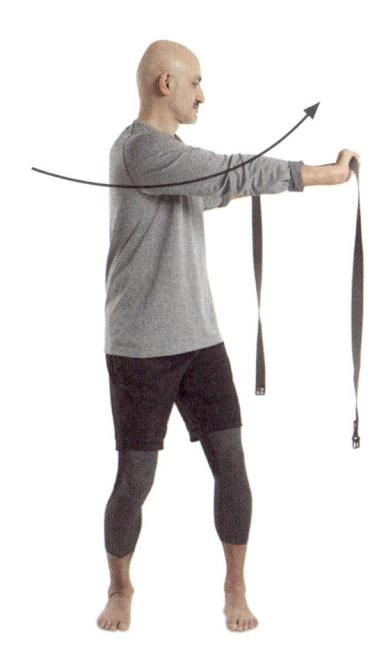

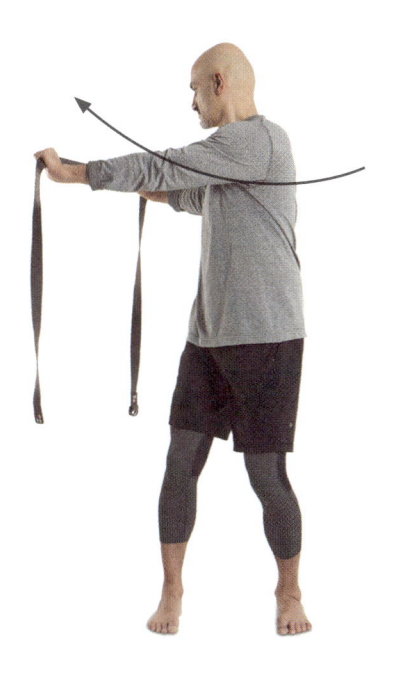

- Hold your strap in front, at chest height, with your palms facing downwards.
- Gently swing your arms over to the left.
- Return to the centre.
- Gently swing your arms over to the right, then return to centre.
- Continue swinging, keeping the movement slow and smooth.
- Breathe in and out as you swing.

REPS: Four on each side.

PLAY: Experiment with lowering the strap to belly height or up to shoulder height.

CHANGE IT UP

If you want it tougher... Try the Advanced version of this Move on page 167.

If you want it more gentle... For a less-strenuous version of this Move, see page 121.

MOVE 6: Shoulder Flossing

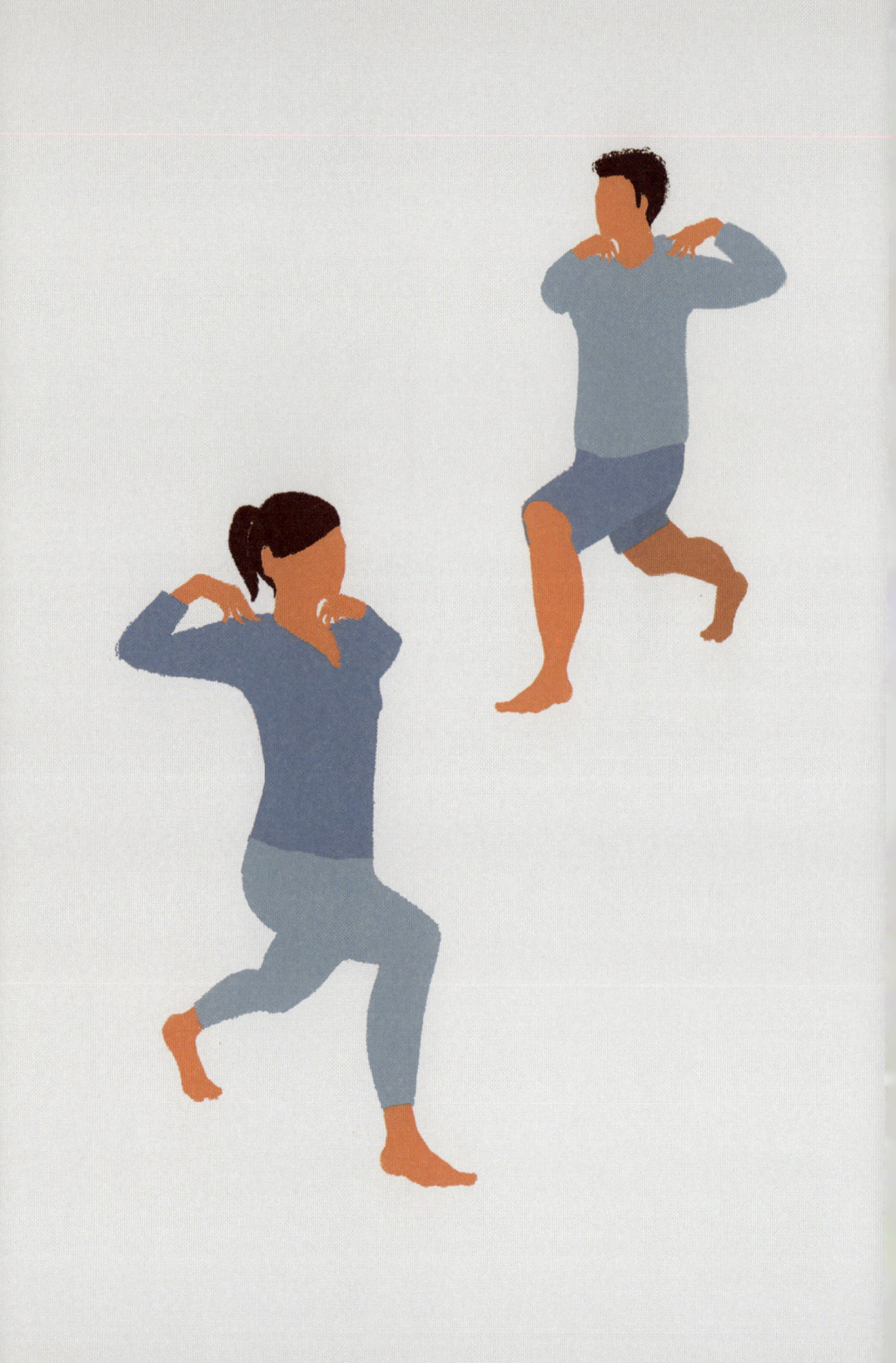

GENTLE MOVES

Life shouldn't always be *push, push, push*. If you expend enough energy at work and want to kick back a little then this is the super-chilled, low-effort way to stay supple.

These Moves, which are simply more gentle and more accessible versions of the six Main Moves, would also suit those who are not keen to clamber up and down to the floor, and anyone who has had time out and needs to ease back into movement.

Some of these 'Moves Lite' use a chair instead of the all fours or cross-legged positions, but still replicate the same rounding, arching and lateral stretches as their Main counterparts, so you won't be missing out.

Gentle Hamstring Releasing uses a strap to let you lie back and access tighter hammies at leisure, with no back strain and also no balance or strength required.

Others take the strap away. For example, Gentle Shoulder Flossing uses strapless soft swaying and circling movements to tease out knotted shoulders.

There may be a host of reasons why Gentle Moves suit your body better. You might be recovering from an injury but still want to maintain a basic level of flexibility. Pushing a joint into its full range of motion at this stage could be unwise. If you simply haven't stretched for a while then this section is a fantastic place to start back on the road to better overall mobility.

However, please don't be confined to this Gentle section if you want to wander. We know that flexibility is joint specific. This means you could have tight hamstrings but pliant shoulders or malleable hips. So, pick and mix Moves from the Main, Gentle and Advanced sections to create a routine perfect for *your* body.

Equipment-wise, you will need a chair and a cotton yoga strap, but an old tie or dressing gown belt is a great strap substitute.

Enjoy your Gentle Moves.

MOVE 1
GENTLE BACK MOBILITY

If you have one of those sensitive backs that needs a little sweet talking to get going then this routine is ideal since it can be done first thing in the morning while still lying in bed, or last thing at night to iron out any kinks. The comforting swaying, hugging and massaging movements release tension, restore mobility and just feel nice. After all, who doesn't enjoy a Snow Angel?

Lying supine (face up) is a great way to assess how your back feels without any strain and is always my foundation point to begin working on overall flexibility. In this relaxed position it is easier to gauge exactly where the back feels tight. Is it the lower back, mid-back or up around the neck or shoulder blades? Or is the restriction lower down in the hips? Or up in the shoulders? It's also a fine excuse to stay in a nice cosy bed for another five minutes.

This sequence mimics most of the Main Back Mobility Move techniques but in a softer way. This might mean keeping your legs bent rather than straight, which can be uncomfortable on the lower back, or resisting pushing to the limit of the stretch and just exploring how far feels good for you.

Maybe there is also a variation of these movements that suits your body better. There are several invitations to explore aspects of the techniques, so look out for the Play sign at the end of Side to Side, Snow Angels and Quarter Clocks. For example, the suggestion in Quarter Clocks is to gradually increase how far round an imaginary clock face you circle your arm. Try to keep your fingertips close to the floor and move in slow motion, breathing in and out as you inch the arm around.

STEP 1

GENTLE BACK MASSAGE

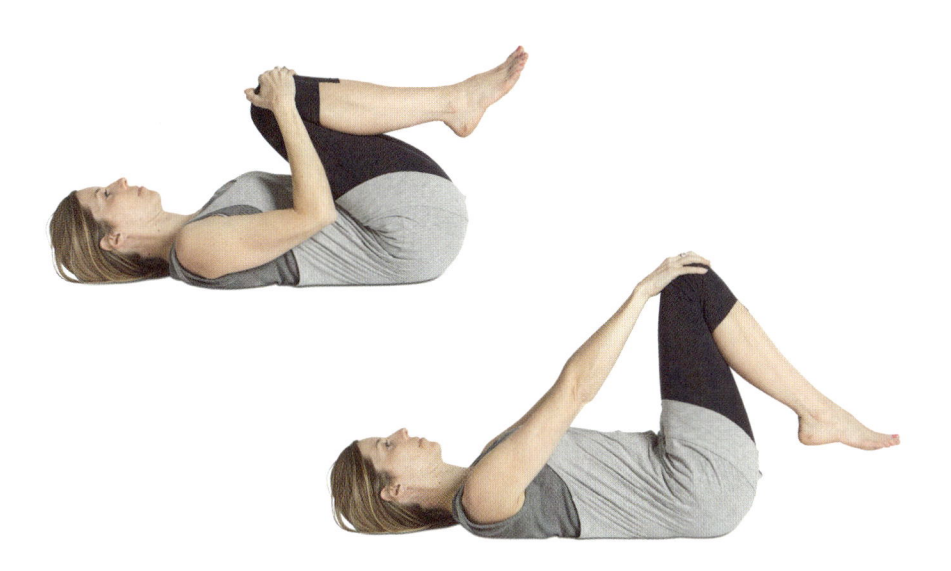

- Lie on your back, placing a cushion under your head if your chin is tilting up.
- Hug both legs into your body and place one hand on each knee.
- As you inhale, move the knees away until the arms straighten.
- As you exhale, hug the legs back into your body.
- Continue, sliding the knees away and drawing them closer.

REPS: Six.

STEP 2

SIMPLE BRIDGES

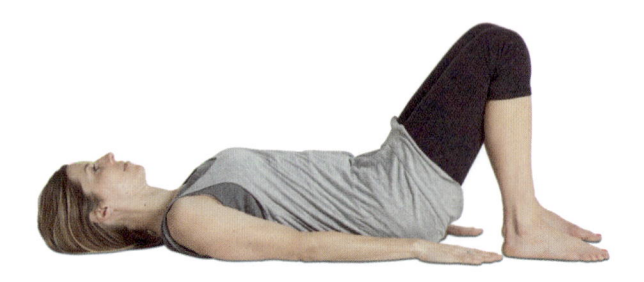

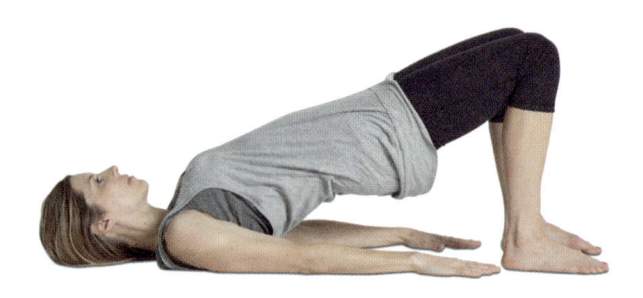

- If you used a cushion for Gentle Back Massage, remove it now.
- Place both arms by your sides, palms facing down.
- As you inhale, lift your hips off the floor, as high as is comfortable.
- As you exhale, lower them to the floor.
- Repeat, slowly lifting and lowering.

REPS: Six.

TIP: Close your eyes as you move, for better body awareness.

STEP 3

GENTLE LEG HUGS

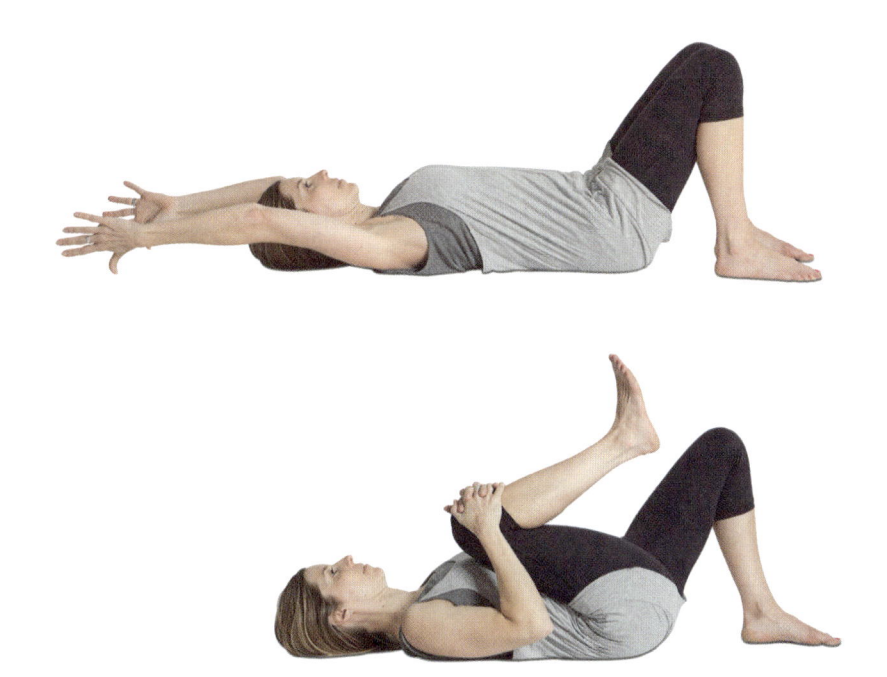

- Keep your legs bent and feet hip-width apart.
- As you inhale, raise both arms above your head.
- As you exhale, hug your right leg into your body
- As you inhale, raise both arms above your head.
- As you exhale, hug your left leg into your body.
- Repeat to complete the reps.

REPS: Six on each side.

STEP 4

SIDE TO SIDE

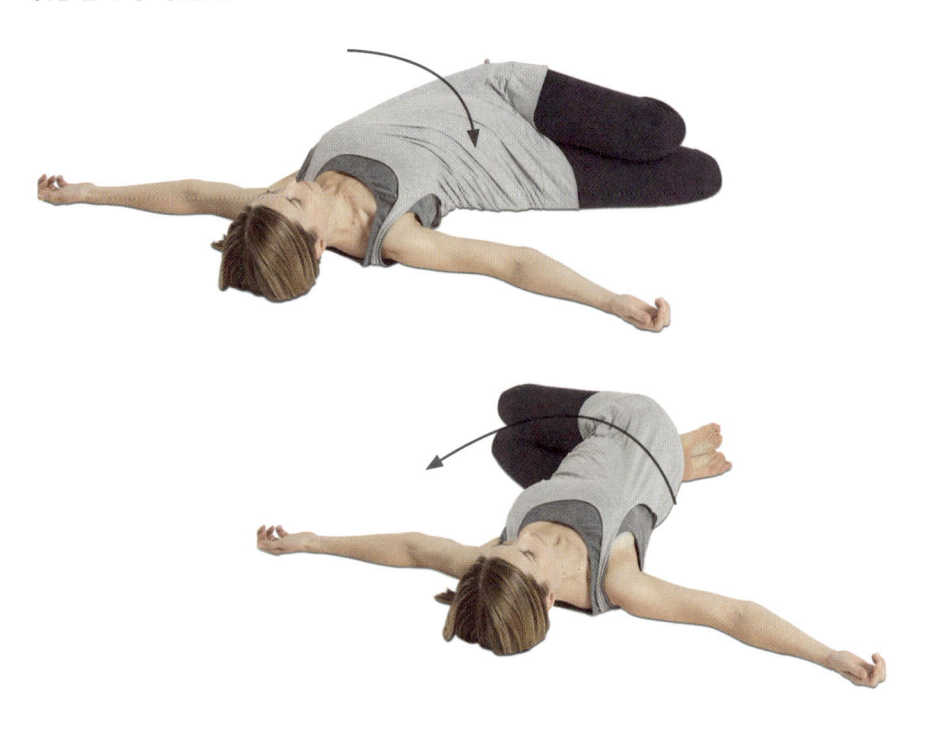

- Keep your legs bent but step your feet together.
- Stretch your arms out to the sides, at shoulder height, palms facing up.
- Exhale and lower both knees down towards the floor to the right.
- Inhale and return the knees to the centre.
- Exhale and lower both knees down towards the floor to the left.
- Inhale and return the knees to the centre.
- Continue to sway the knees slowly from side to side to complete the reps.

REPS: Four on each side.

PLAY: Gradually drop your knees a little lower each time you sway them to the side.

STEP 5

SNOW ANGELS

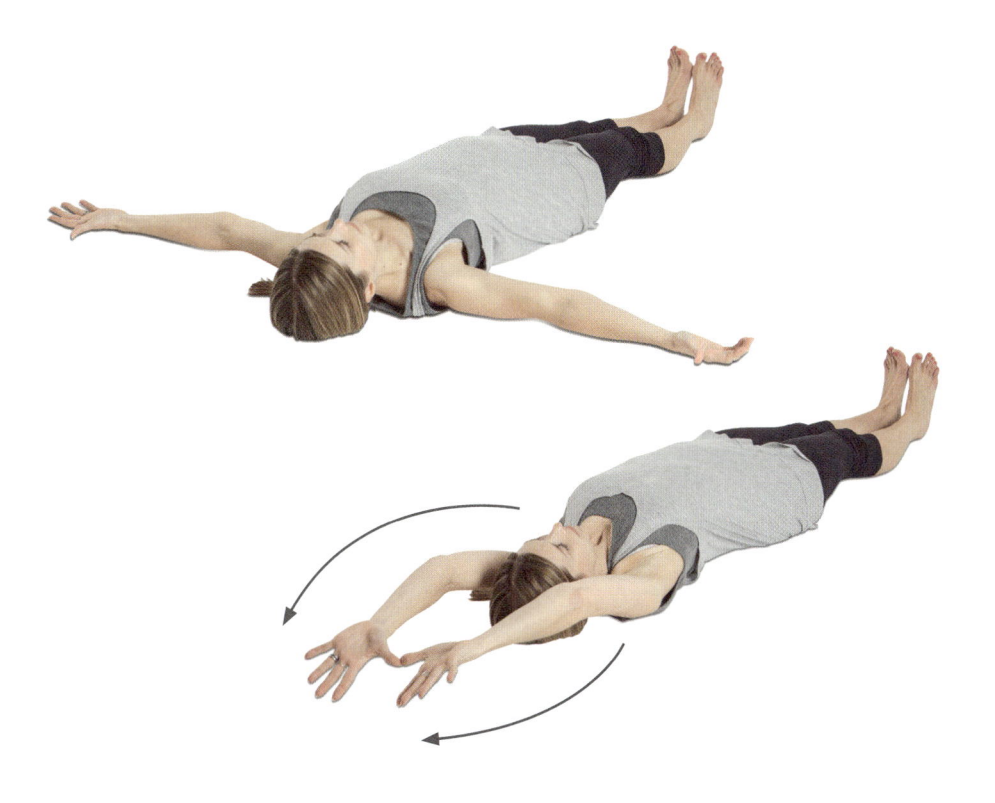

- Keep your legs bent but move your feet hip-width apart, or straighten your legs.
- Stretch your arms out at shoulder height, palms facing up.
- Lift both arms so that they hover just off the floor (or higher if the shoulders are stiff).
- As you inhale, sweep both arms overhead until the thumbs touch.
- As you exhale, return them to shoulder height.
- Repeat to complete the reps.

REPS: Four–six.

PLAY: Aim to keep your arms as close to the floor as possible.

MOVE 1: Gentle Back Mobility

STEP 6
QUARTER CLOCKS

Roll on to your right side with your legs bent into a 90-degree position.

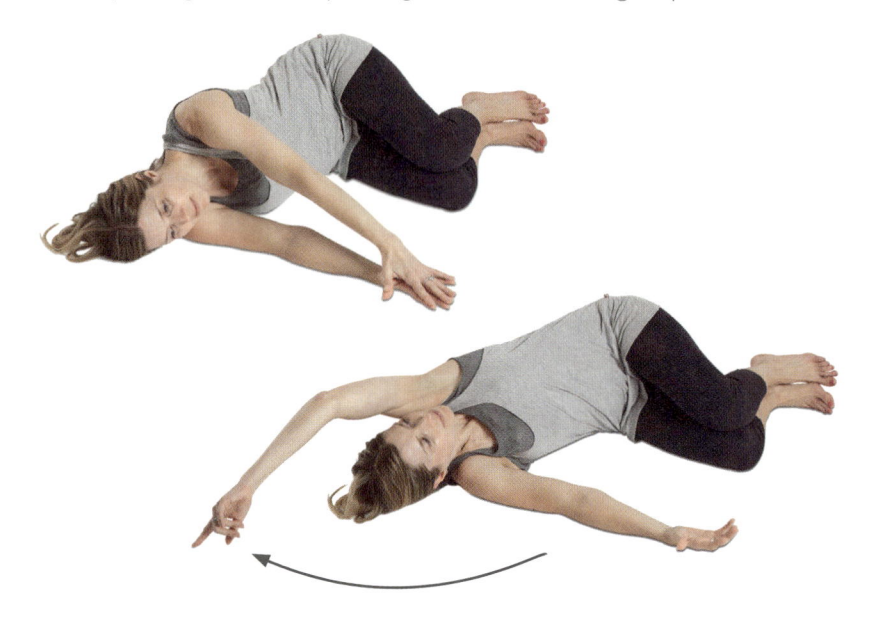

- Straighten your arms and place your palms together.
- As you inhale, sweep your left arm up above, or just past, your head, as if drawing a quarter of a circle.
- As you exhale, bring your palms back together again.
- Continue to move, sweeping the arm up and back.
- Roll on to your left side and sweep your right arm up and down in the same way.

REPS: Six on each side.

PLAY: Move the arm a little further around the clock face each time, increasing it from 15 minutes to 20, 25 and so on. Alternatively, feel free to circle the arm all the way around.

CHANGE IT UP

If you want it tougher...
Try the Advanced version of this Move on page 132.

MOVE 2
GENTLE CAT PLAY

Don't want to get down on all fours? No problem. Here's a more accessible version of Cat Play with all the same feline-inspired, decompressing and releasing moves for the back, neck and shoulders, but done from the comfort of a seat. So, the next time your back feels a little stiff, just pull up a chair and play.

Cat Play is the back-focused sequence to pick if you find it difficult to get up and down from the floor, as it is completely chair-based.

We start the sequence by playing with the two spinal movements that form the yoga flow Cat Stretch – flexion and extension (rounding and arching). The idea is to alternate between the two opposing movements to warm up the back and then feed in lateral (side) stretching and rotation.

The seated element means that this Move would also work well in the office to release the tension that can creep in around the lower back or shoulders after sitting with the back in a fixed flexed position.

Pick a simple, sturdy chair and perch with a straight back on the edge of it. Ideally your legs should form a right-angle shape if both feet are planted hip-width apart on the floor.

This 'sitting tall' position is our foundation posture for beginning to explore all the movements of the spine that keep a back happy and healthy. This includes loosening up the thoracic or mid-back through the tiny rotational movement featured in step 5, Thoracic Twist.

> **MOVE IT ON:** If you have the time, add two more chair-based Moves from this Gentle section of the book – Gentle Unstick the Hips and Gentle Hamstring Releasing – to create more of a whole-body movement routine.

TIP: MOVE SLOWLY AND IN A CAT-LIKE FASHION TO AVOID ANY JARRING MOVEMENTS.

STEP 1

CAT STRETCH

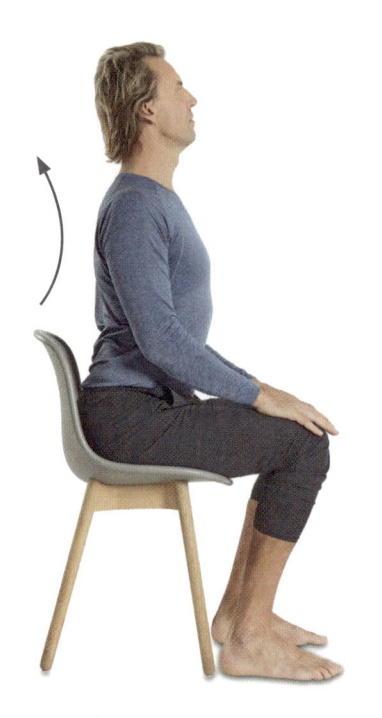

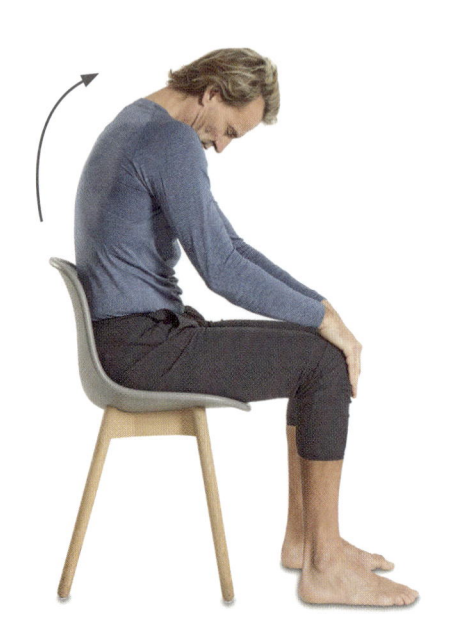

- Sit tall with one hand on each thigh.
- Inhale, lift your chest and chin and draw back your shoulders.
- Exhale, round or flex your back and tuck in your tailbone.
- Continue, inhaling to lift your chest and exhaling to flex your back.

REPS: Six.

STEP 2

SIDE STRETCH

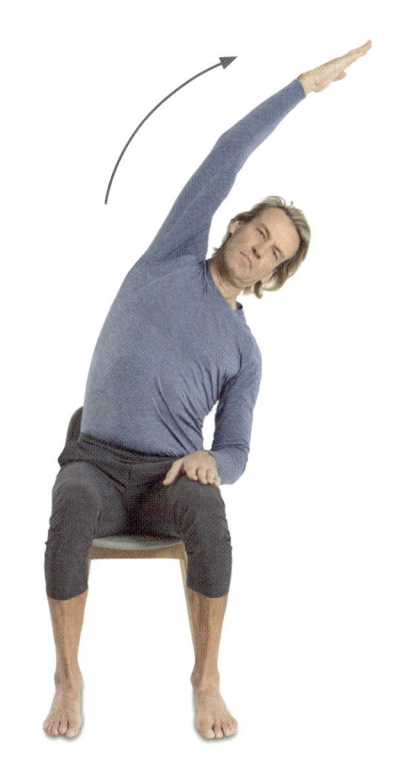

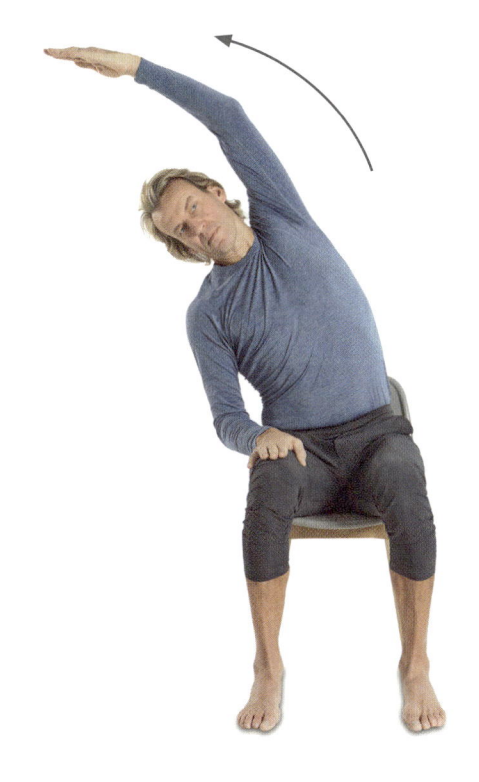

- Place your right hand on your right thigh.
- Reach your left arm up but keep it slightly bent and relaxed.
- Exhale and lean over to the right.
- Inhale and return to centre.
- Place you left hand on your left thigh.
- Reach your right arm up.
- Exhale and lean over to the left.
- Continue, inhaling to the centre and exhaling over to the side.

REPS: Three on each side.

MOVE 2: Gentle Cat Play

STEP 3

THUMBS UP

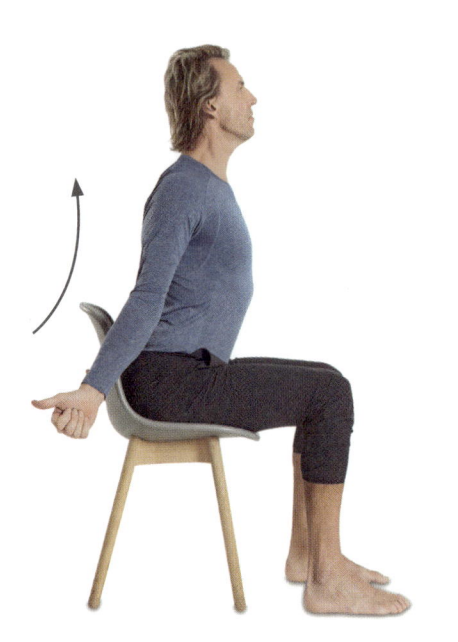

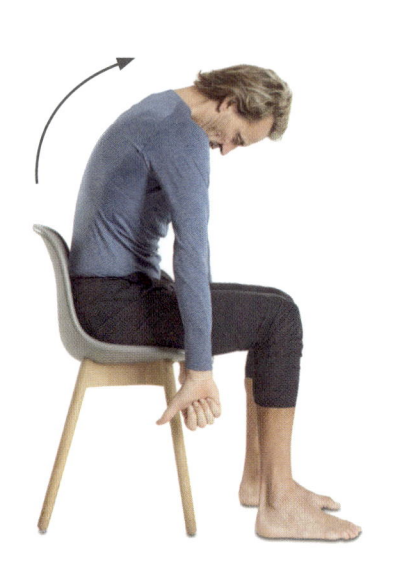

- Take your arms by your side and make a 'thumbs up' hand position.
- As you inhale, lift your chest and point your thumbs back so your palms face upwards.
- As you exhale, let your shoulders round as you point your thumbs down.
- Continue to switch between the two movements, alternately pointing the thumbs up and down.

REPS: Six.

STEP 4

CHAIR FLOW

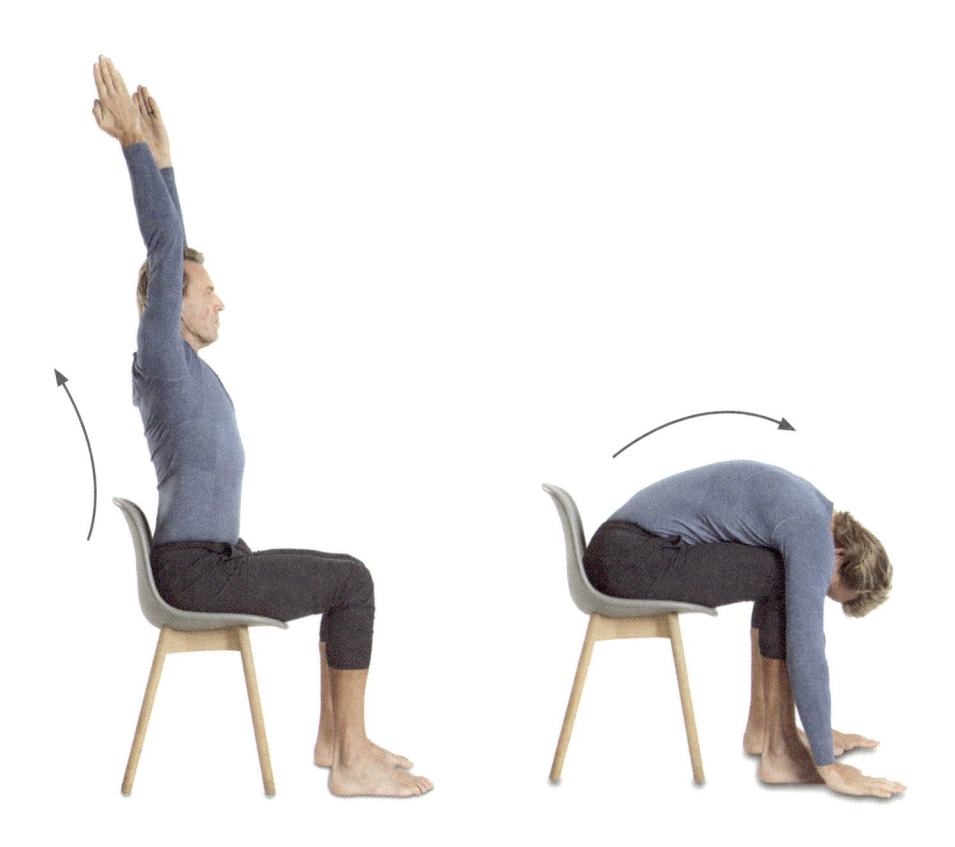

- Inhale and raise both arms up above your head. Lift your chin slightly.
- Exhale and fold forwards, flexing the back. Bend your arms and place your hands on your thighs. If this is easy, drop your hands down to touch your feet as you fold forwards.
- Continue to reach up and fold forwards.

REPS: Four.

MOVE 2: Gentle Cat Play

STEP 5

THORACIC TWIST

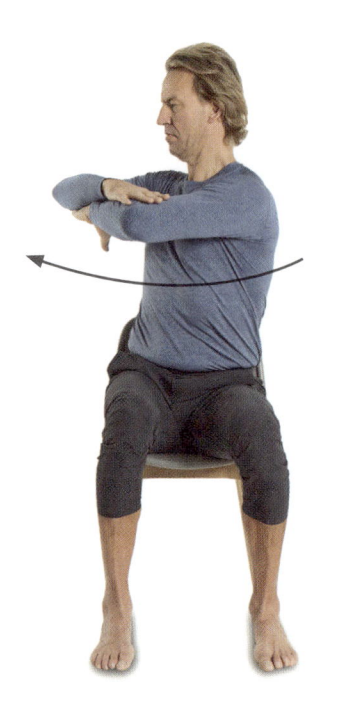

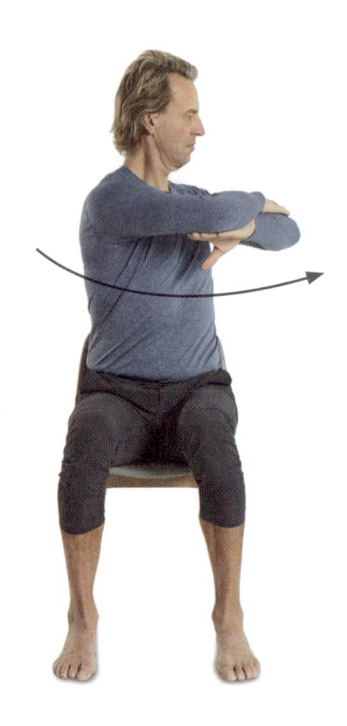

- Cross your arms and lift them so they are at chest height.
- Slowly rotate your torso and arms from side to side.
- Move the arms and torso together as if they are one unit and let the head turn with the torso.
- Continue with this small movement, breathing in and out as you rotate.

REPS: Move slowly for 10–20 seconds.

PLAY: We are aiming to isolate the mid-spine with this tiny movement so try not to turn your head or swing your arms ahead of your torso. Less is more!

STEP 6

TURNS, TIPS AND ROLLS

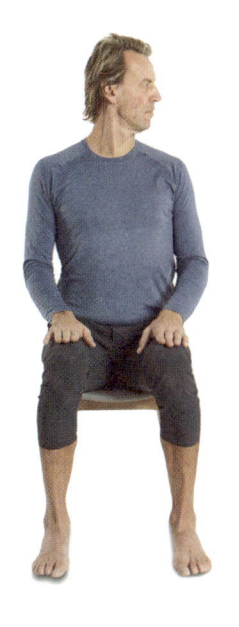

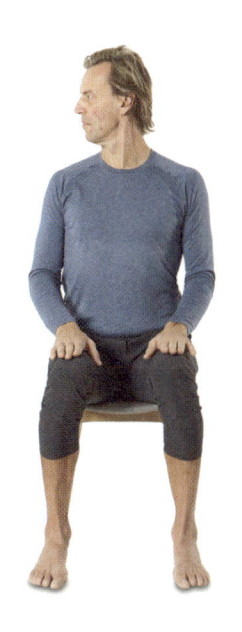

- Sit tall but relax your shoulders.
- Turn your head to the right.
- Turn your head to the left.
- Tip your right ear to your right shoulder
- Tip your left ear to your left shoulder.
- Drop the head down and roll it slowly in a semicircle. Avoid tipping the head back.
- Breathe slowly in and out as you move.

REPS: Move slowly for 20 seconds or longer.

PLAY: Mix up any of these movements or stick with the one you prefer. Close your eyes as you move and hunt for tight spots.

MOVE 2: Gentle Cat Play

MOVE 3
GENTLE UNSTICK THE HIPS

Having a busy office job is no excuse for letting those hips seize up. With a little crafty circling and sweeping it is possible to retain hip mobility throughout the nine-to-five and beyond. Most of these friendly movements can be done without leaving your seat, and colleagues will never know you are undertaking secret hip flexibility training.

We stick with the chair for this Gentle hip flexibility routine. This makes it a handy sequence for two groups of people:

First, those who have a desk job but are still keen to maintain hip movement to avoid lower back issues (tight hips are a contributor to lower back problems).

Second, those who just find it easier mobility-wise to use a chair rather than manoeuvring up and down to the floor.

There are others who might favour this version of Unstick the Hips over the Main sequence simply because they find sitting cross-legged uncomfortable or impossible. So, if you haven't sat this way since junior school, just grab a chair instead. You won't be missing out; the mechanics of the movements are very similar in both Moves.

We start by circling each hip, do some lateral flexion (side bending) to stretch the outer hip, and follow this with a few 'glute' or buttock stretches. We then mix in a lunge and end with a wider-legged movement to replace that cross-legged stance. Just ignore any odd looks from work colleagues!

Some of these movements can visibly show a hip flexibility imbalance, particularly 90 Leans. On the tighter side the knee will be higher up, or more reluctant to drop down, and could be closer to your body. If one hip is visibly stiffer, hold the lean forwards for 10–20 seconds after completing your reps.

Take note: if you have had a hip replacement surgery please seek your surgeon's advice. Movements such as hip flexion beyond 90 degrees and the external hip rotation in 90 Leans are not advised for a certain period of time after surgery.

STEP 1

HIP CIRCLING

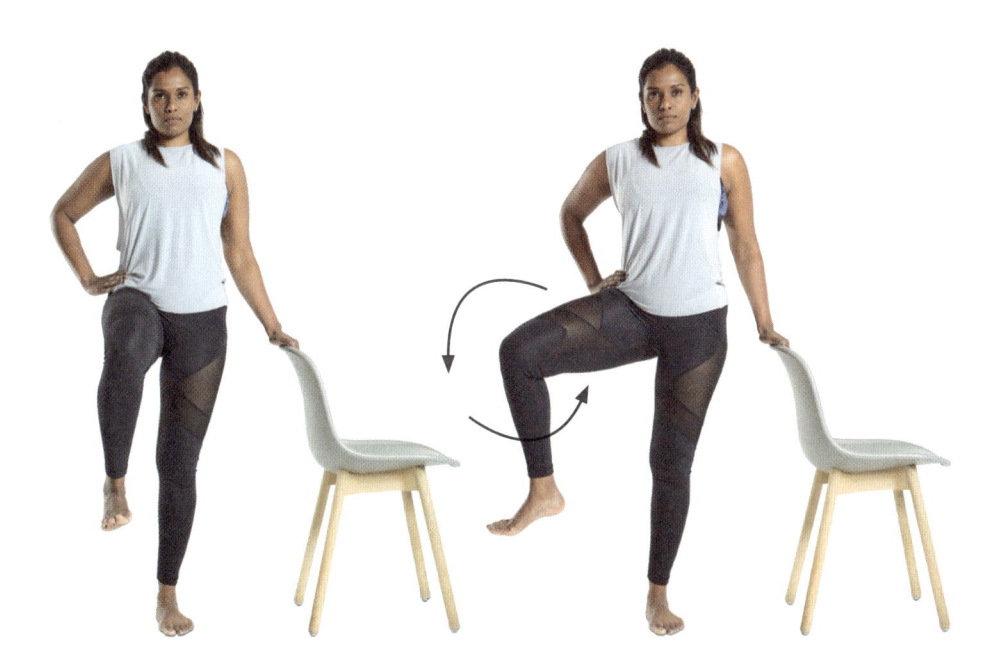

- Stand tall behind your chair. Turn to the side and place your left hand on the back of the seat for balance.

- Lift your right knee up and begin to make a circular motion with the knee by taking it out to the right, drawing it back and sweeping it through to the start position. Keep the knee high all the way around the circle.

- Continue to circle, breathing in and out as you move.

- Complete the reps, then switch legs.

REPS: Six on each side.

PLAY: Try taking your hand off the chair to challenge your balance.

MOVE 3: Gentle Unstick the Hips

STEP 2

SIDE SWEEPS

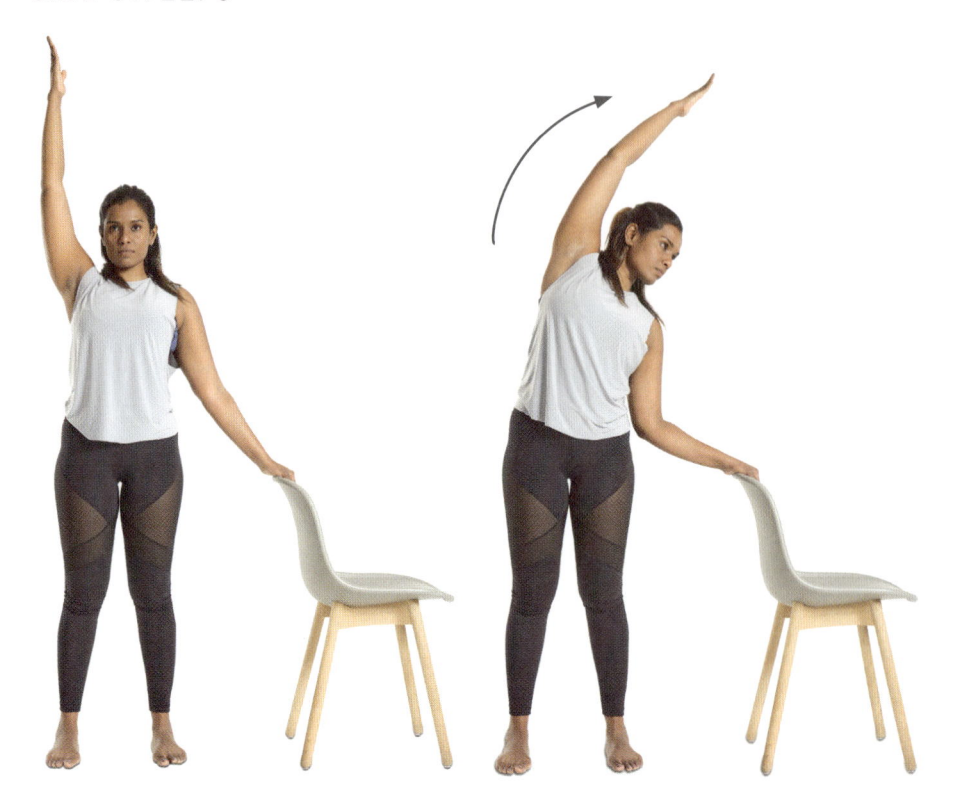

- Stay standing behind the chair with your left hand on the back of the chair for balance.
- Reach your right arm up.
- Exhale, lean towards the chair and sweep your right arm over by your head.
- Inhale and return to centre, reaching your right arm up.
- Continue with the movement. Inhale to stand and exhale to lean.
- Complete the reps. Switch sides by turning to face the other way.

REPS: Four–six on each side.

PLAY: To deepen the side stretch, step your right leg across your left.

96 MOVE

STEP 3

BUTTERFLY FOLDS

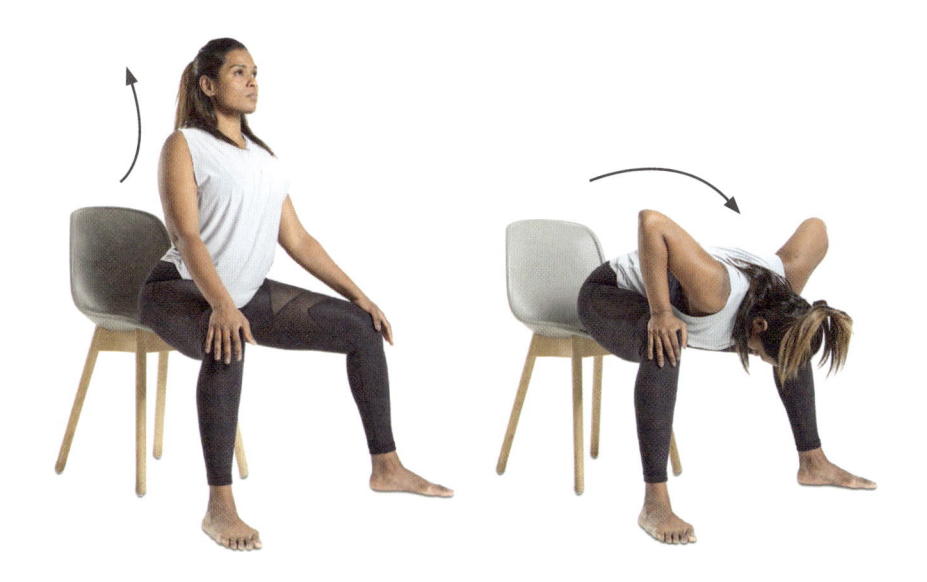

- Sit on the edge of the chair with your feet wide and your toes turned slightly outwards. Rest your hands on your thighs.
- Inhale to sit tall with a straight back.
- Exhale to fold over your legs by bending your arms and rounding or flexing your back.
- Continue to complete the reps.

REPS: Five.

PLAY: Fold lower by dropping your fingertips down to the floor. Or stay here, cross your arms and hang still.

STEP 4

90 LEANS

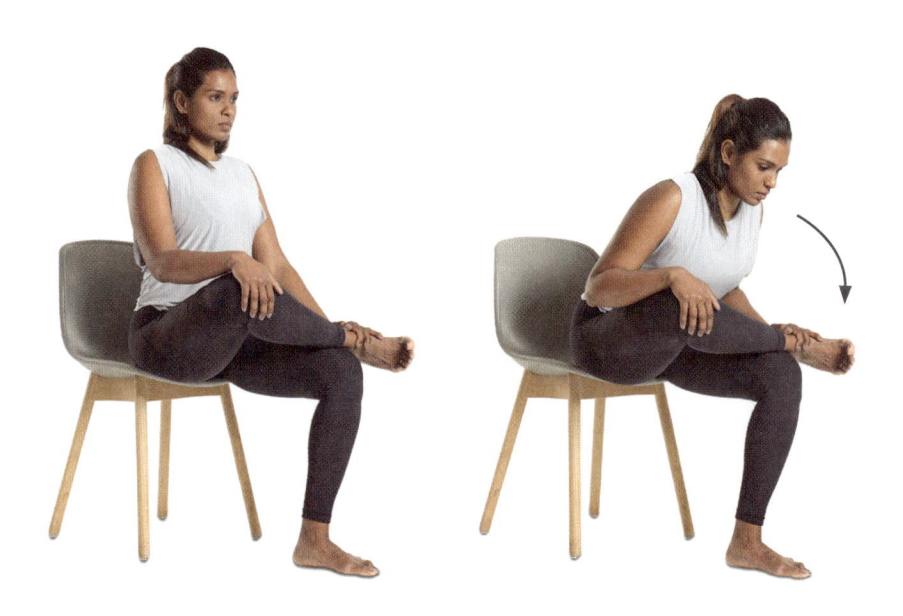

- Bend your right leg, turn your knee out and place your right ankle on top of your left thigh so the leg forms a 90-degree angle
- Sit tall and rest your hands on your right leg.
- Inhale here. As you exhale, lean forwards, keeping a straight back.
- Inhale to sit back up.
- Continue to sit up and fold forwards to complete the reps, then switch legs.

REPS: Six–eight on each side.

PLAY: Pause the 90 Lean and hold for 20 seconds if one hip feels stiffer than the other.

STEP 5

LUNGE DROPS

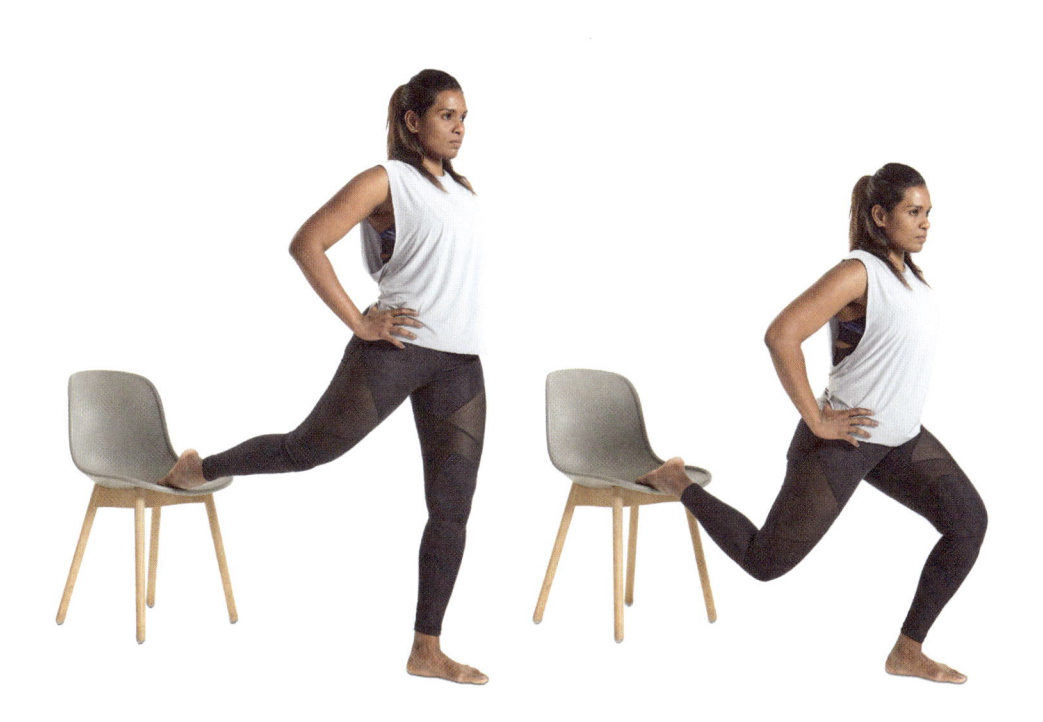

- Stand in front of the chair with your back to it.
- Rest the front of your right foot on the chair seat and stand tall with your hands on your hips to create the lunge start position.
- Tuck in your hips, bend your standing leg and dip down a little into a lunge, taking care not to strain your front knee.
- Inhale to stand up and exhale to dip down.
- Complete the reps, then switch legs.

REPS: Six on each side.

STEP 6

HUG AND TURN

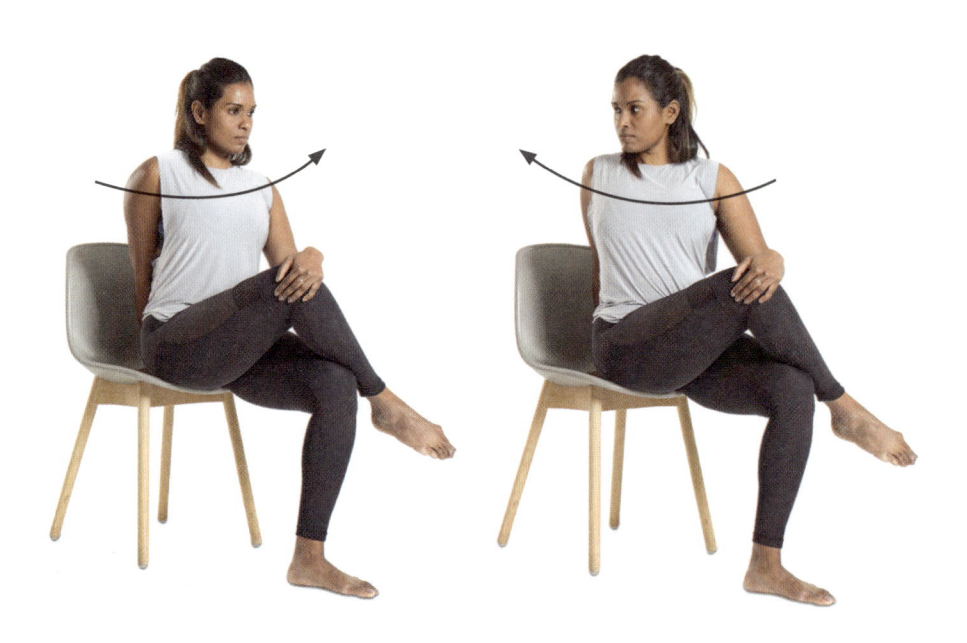

- Sit tall on the edge of the chair.
- Cross your legs, placing your right leg on top.
- Place your left hand on your right knee and your right hand behind your back.
- Exhale and rotate your head and shoulders to the right.
- Inhale and return to the start position.
- Complete the reps, then switch sides.

REPS: Four on each side.

PLAY: For a harder version, hug the top leg into the body.

CHANGE IT UP

If you want it tougher...
Try the Advanced version of this Move on page 146.

MOVE 4
GENTLE LUNGE FLOW

Ignore the strange looks and break into a spontaneous lunge – your body will thank you! Lunging is a fantastic way to unravel the hunched or flexed position we use when sitting, slouching or texting, by opening it into extension. Lunges also help prevent lower backache. This is a more accessible version of the Lunge Flow to suit anyone and everyone who feels a little 'crunched'.

This Move mirrors the basic Lunge Flow but with no need to drop the back knee all the way down to the floor. This makes it perfect for a bit of spontaneous stretching. The sequence also works well if your hips are feeling a bit stiffer than normal, perhaps post run or first thing in the morning when the legs and hips need some oiling to get lubricated.

Want to make your lunge count? There are a few things to consider:

First, tuck in your backside and keep it locked in position until you reach the final step. This is the most effective way to stretch the hip flexors (iliopsoas muscles) at the front of the hip.

Second, don't position the back foot directly behind the front in your basic lunge position as this makes it wobbly, a bit like standing on a tightrope. Imagine instead that you are standing on train tracks with your feet placed wider apart.

Finally, spread your toes. This will improve balance, which you will need a good sense of when we start waving our arms around. If you still feel unstable, grab a chair and place it by your side. You can hold the back of the chair with one hand while you sweep the other arm back and forth.

> Start with your right leg forwards and move through the entire flow, then repeat the sequence with the left foot in front.

TIP: KEEP YOUR FRONT KNEE POSITIONED ABOVE OR JUST BEHIND YOUR ANKLE IN THE LUNGE.

STEP 1

SLIDING

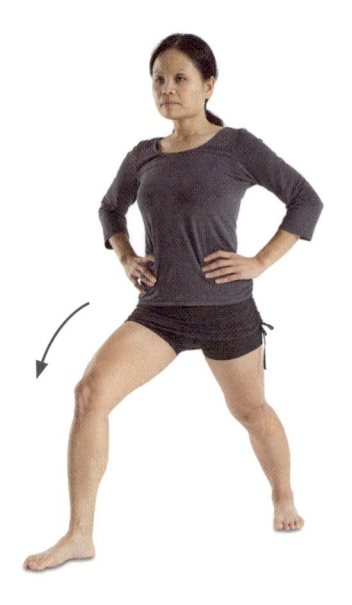

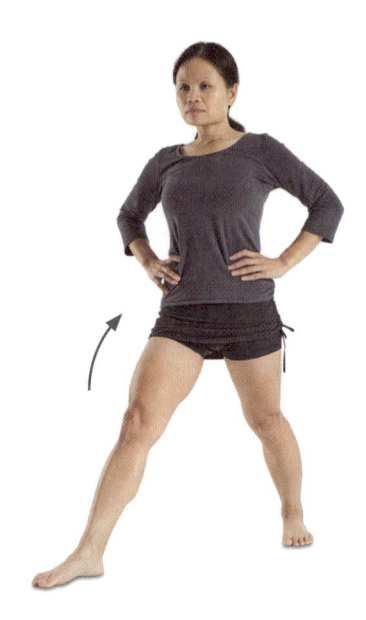

- Stand with your feet hip-width apart and your hands on your hips.
- Step your left foot back, keeping the feet parallel.
- Tuck in your backside.
- Exhale and bend your front leg to move into the lunge, ensuring that the front knee is either above or behind the front ankle.
- Inhale and straighten your front leg to rise back up.
- Continue to slide in and out of the lunge, exhaling into it and inhaling to rise back up.

REPS: Four

STEP 2

ELBOW CIRCLING

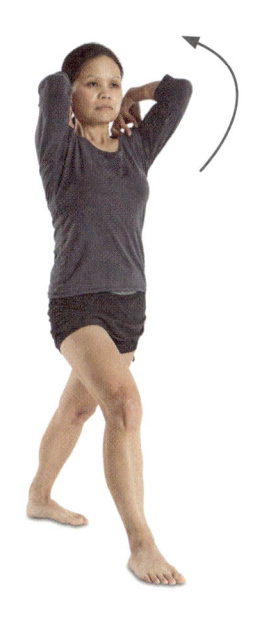

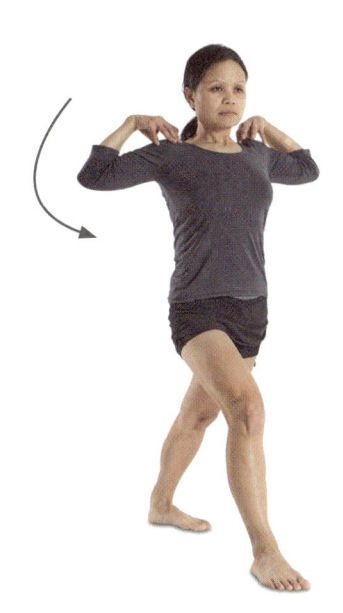

- Hold the lunge position with the front leg bent.
- Lift your upper body.
- Place both hands lightly on top of your shoulders.
- Make slow circles with both elbows, breathing evenly.

REPS: Six, moving forwards or backwards.

MOVE 4: Gentle Lunge Flow

STEP 3

ELBOW POINTING

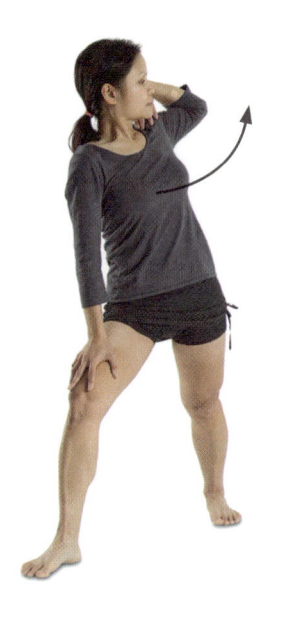

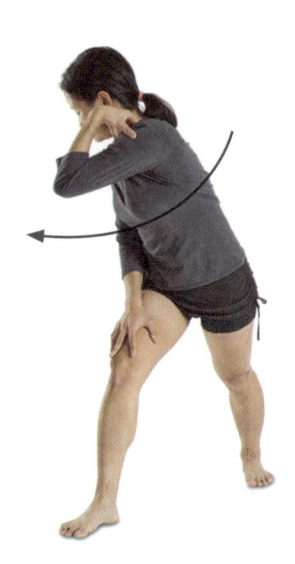

- Keep your left hand on your left shoulder. Drop your right hand to rest on your right thigh.
- As you inhale, point the left elbow behind you.
- As you exhale, sweep the elbow past your right leg and point it down to the floor.
- Repeat, pointing back and down.

REPS: Four

STEP 4

LUNGE WAVING

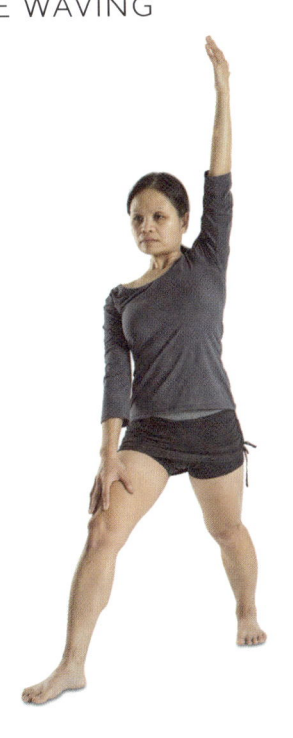

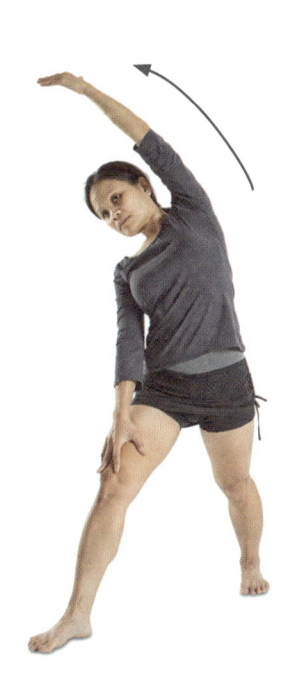

- Reach your left arm up above your head. Inhale here.
- As you exhale, sweep your left arm over to the right.
- Repeat, inhaling to the centre and exhaling over.

REPS: Four

STEP 5

LUNGE TWISTING

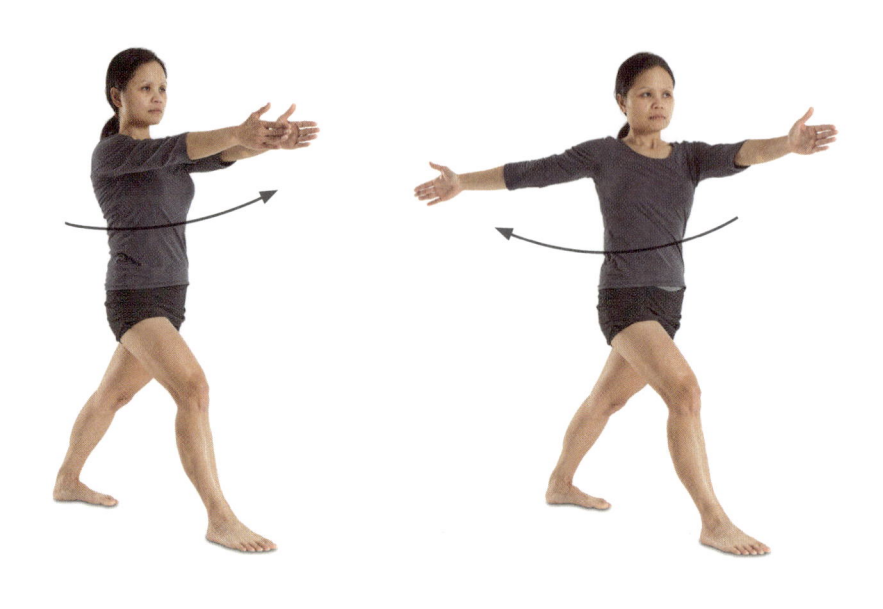

- Reach both arms forwards at chest height with your palms facinging each other.
- As you inhale, sweep your right arm back.
- As you exhale, return it to the start position.
- As you inhale, sweep your left arm back.
- As you exhale, return it to the start position.
- Continue to move smoothly from side to side to complete the reps.

REPS: Four

PLAY: Turn your head as you sweep each arm to challenge your balance.

STEP 6

SIDE LUNGING

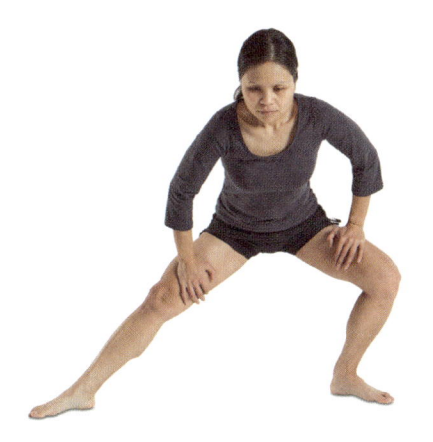

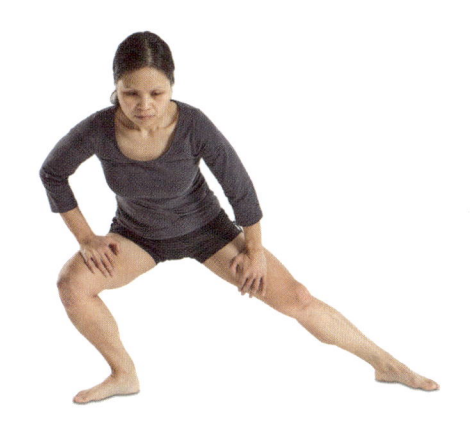

- Move your feet wide apart and turn your toes slightly outwards.
- Place your hands on your thighs and lean slightly forwards, keeping your back straight and core engaged.
- Exhale, bend your left leg and straighten your right leg. Ensure that your left knee does not bend too deeply and that the knee tracks in line with the left foot.
- Inhale and return to the centre.
- Exhale, bend your right leg and straighten your left leg.
- Inhale to return to the centre.
- Continue to flow slowly from side to side to complete the reps.

REPS: Four–six

CHANGE IT UP

If you want it tougher...
Try the Advanced version of this Move on page 153.

MOVE 4: Gentle Lunge Flow

MOVE 5
GENTLE HAMSTRING RELEASING

Lie back and think of your hammies in this relaxed version of the Hamstring Releasing Move. The tricky standing and balancing techniques have gone, replaced by the much more fun-sounding Boat Rowing, Kite Flying and Windscreen Wiping, all done lying flat on your back. So now there's no excuse not to stretch your hamstrings.

You might notice that the Main, Advanced and Gentle Moves in this book are visually similar – just harder or easier versions of the same movements. However, this particular routine breaks the mould by looking very different from its Main and Hard counterparts. For the Gentle version, we lie face-up the floor, grab a strap and hook it around the leg. The reason for this is because this is the best way to isolate the hamstrings without worrying about factors such as balance or strength – distractions that we can do without.

It's also easy to confuse a stiff back with tight hamstrings. For example, when you sit on the floor, straighten your legs and try to touch your toes, is it a restriction in your lower back or your hamstrings that stops you? It can be hard to tell. Here, we take the back out of the equation (by lying on it) to concentrate solely on those rope-like muscles behind the thigh.

Have fun with your Boat Rowing and Kite Flying but remember to go easy. Hamstrings are sensitive to being stretched too hard and fast so go slowly and glide in and out of the reps. Think about coming to the 'edge' of the stretch and then moving out again as you perform your reps, keeping the breathing deep.

Also, please feel no pressure to lock the leg straight when sitting in Boat Rowing or lying down. This is a golden rule with hamstring stretching. You will *still* be stretching your hammies with a bent leg and it will probably feel a lot better.

If your hamstrings are particularly tight, end this sequence by returning to the Kite Flying start position and hold the stretch for 30–60 seconds.

You will need a cotton yoga strap (or dressing gown belt or old tie) and enough room to lie down and wave your leg around.

TIP: DON'T LOCK THE LEG STRAIGHT IF THE HAMSTRINGS FEEL TIGHT.

STEP 1

BOAT ROWING

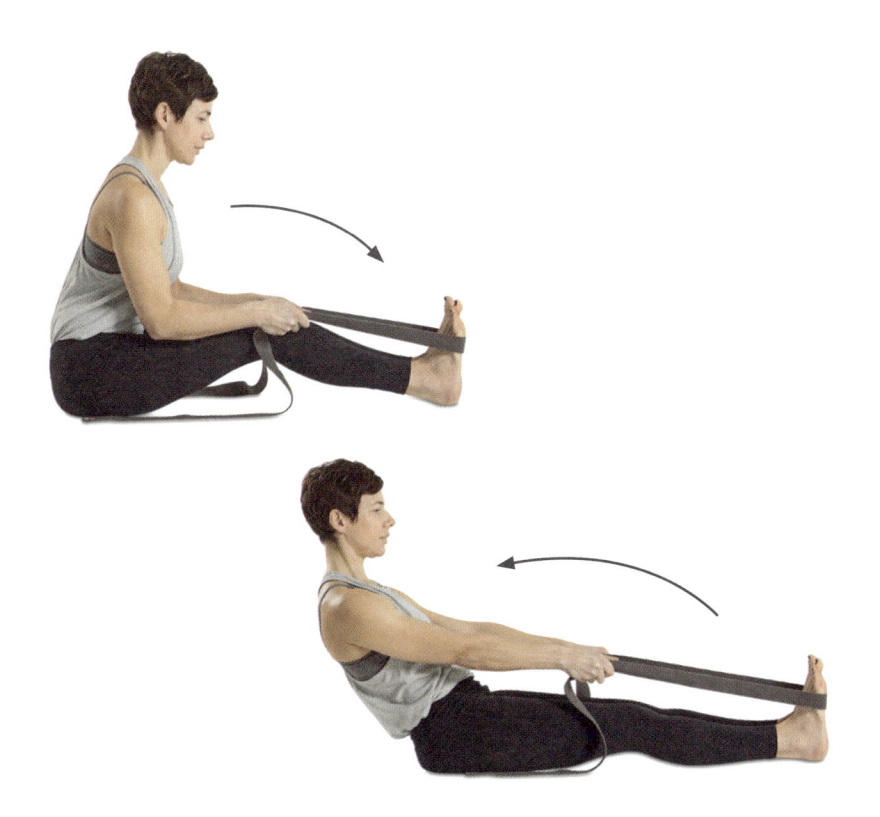

- Sit with a straight back with your legs stretched out in front of you. Bend your legs a little if it's hard to sit tall.
- Hook a strap loosely around your feet and hold on to both parts of the strap.
- As you inhale, tip forwards until you feel the start of a hamstring stretch.
- As you exhale, lean back until you feel the core engage.
- Continue, leaning slowly forwards and back to complete the reps, keeping the back straight.

REPS: Six–eight.

MOVE 5: Gentle Hamstring Releasing

STEP 2

ROTATE AND REACH

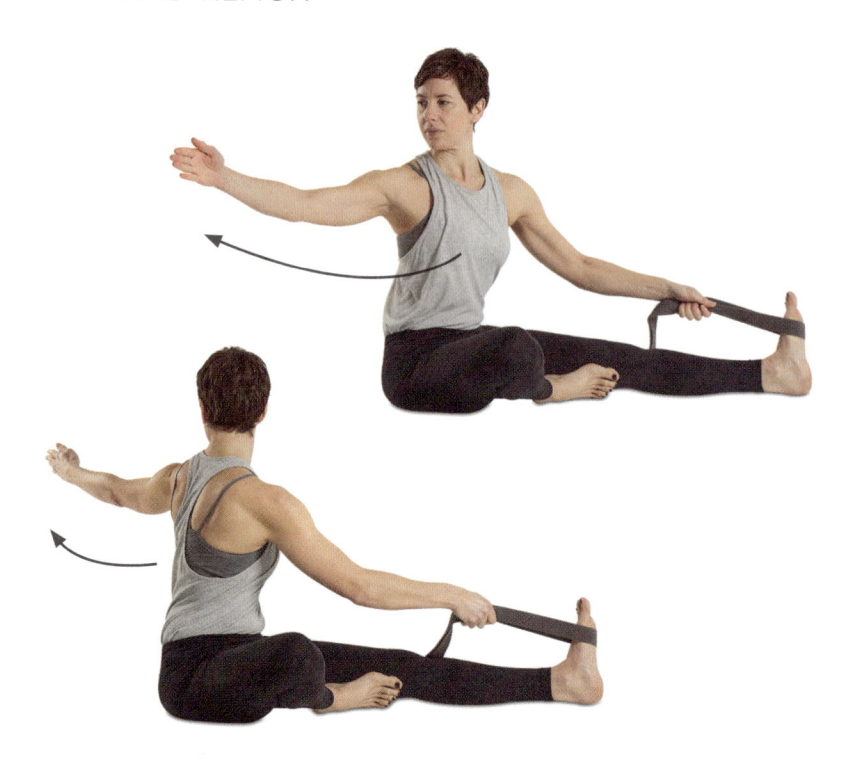

- Sit tall. Bend your right leg and place the sole of your right foot on the inside of your left thigh.
- Hold both parts of the strap with your left hand. Inhale and sweep the right arm behind you.
- Exhale, return it and grab the strap again.
- Inhale, sweep the left arm behind you, then exhale to return it and hold the strap.
- Continue to switch arms, inhaling as you reach back and exhaling to return the arm.
- Complete the reps, then switch legs by bending the left leg and placing the sole of your left foot on the inside of your right thigh.

REPS: Four on each side.

STEP 3

SLOW-MOTION ROLL

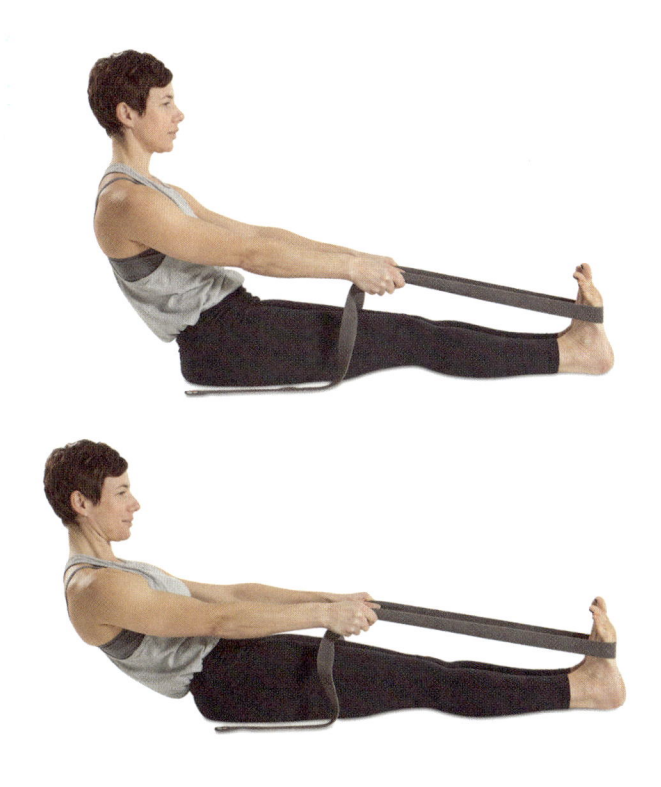

- Loop the strap back around both feet, holding on to the strap with both hands.
- Tuck in your chin and roll down slowly to the floor, letting the strap run slowly through your hands.
- Try to lay the spine down in sections: lower back, mid-back and upper back.

REPS: Just perform one slow-motion roll down.

MOVE 5: Gentle Hamstring Releasing

STEP 4

KITE FLYING

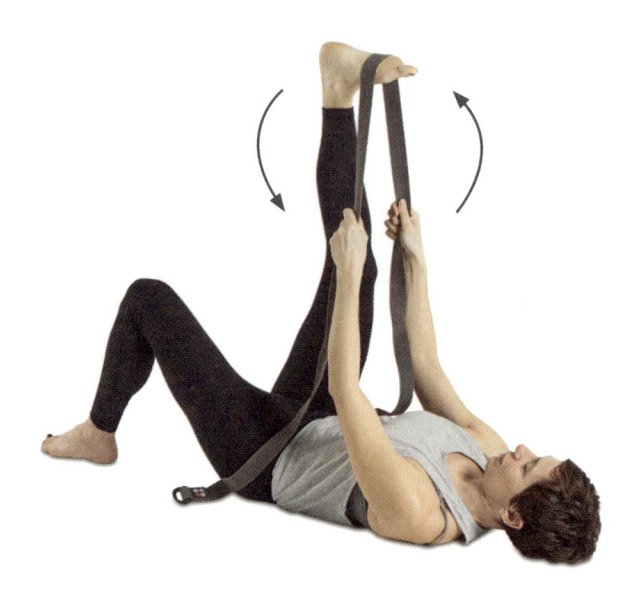

- Bend your left leg and place your foot on the floor.
- Loop the strap around your right foot and straighten your leg up towards the ceiling. Bend the knee if the hamstring feels tight.
- Hold one piece of the strap in each hand and begin to sway the leg slowly around in circles or a figure-of-eight shape. Experiment with different movements but work slowly, breathing in and out through the nose.

REPS: Just continue for a minute or more.

PLAY: Swish the leg from side to side, keep it straight, lower it to the floor and pull it back up until you feel the start of a hamstring stretch. Tip the leg out to the right. Notice where it feels tightest: hamstrings, inner thigh or outer hip.

STEP 5

BEND AND EXTEND

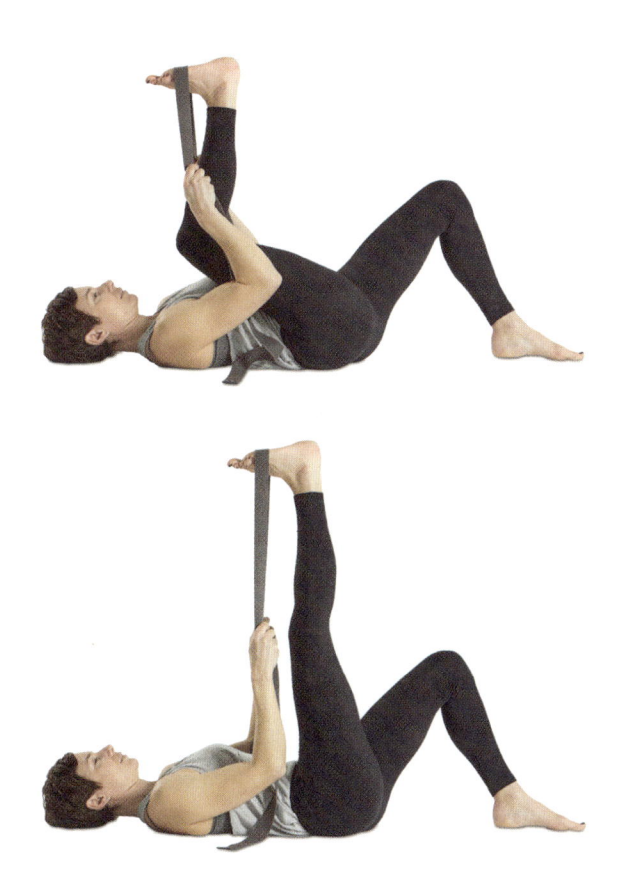

- Return the right leg to the Kite Flying start position.
- Bend it deeply so that the thigh moves towards the belly.
- Straighten it as you move it away.
- Continue to bend and straighten, moving slowly and smoothly.
- Complete the reps, then switch legs.

REPS: Four on each side.

STEP 6

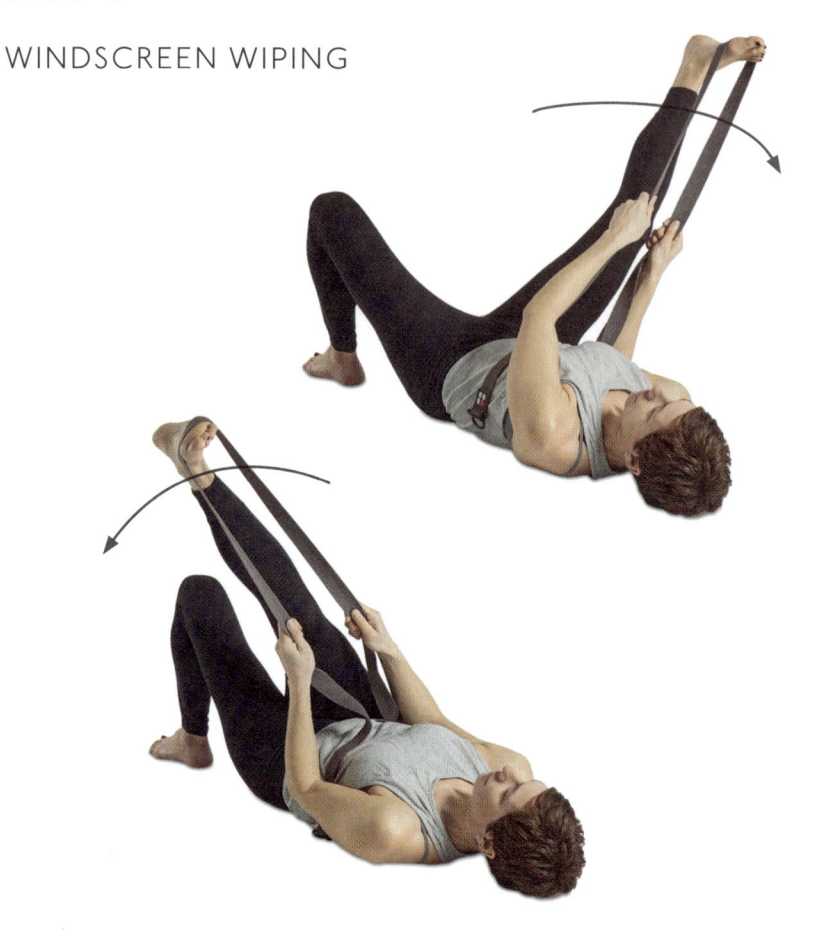

WINDSCREEN WIPING

- Stay with the right leg.
- Hold on to both parts of the strap with both hands.
- As you exhale, swing your right leg over the body to the left side.
- As you inhale, return it to the centre.
- Complete the reps, then switch legs.

REPS: Four on each side.

MOVE 6
GENTLE SHOULDER FLOSSING

They say 'motion is lotion' – the body's ligaments, muscles and tendons need to regularly move through their range of motion to feel good and stay supple. These simple lubricating movements can be done anywhere and act like a balm, soothing tired, stiff shoulder and upper back muscles.

The obvious difference here to the Main Shoulder Flossing Move is the lack of a strap as a stretching aid. Instead, here we focus on very simple lubricating movements for the joint, without any gripping or straining. The idea is to maintain the mobility of the naturally flexible shoulders by systematically loosening up all the surrounding muscle groups with small, repetitive movements.

This type of motion is also thought to release adhesions or knotted areas of the fascia, the thin layer of connective tissue that envelops all our muscles. As we get older our joints also produce less synovial fluid, the joint's natural lubricating fluid, so it becomes even more important to regularly give the shoulders a mobility workout to maintain flexibility.

The plan is to ease these joints through basic flexion, extension and rotational moves without pushing too deep – sometimes, 'less is more'. Simple shoulder rolling feels great whatever your level of shoulder flexibility, especially if done with the eyes closed.

Due to its softer approach this Move might suit people with reduced shoulder mobility or those with tight neck or shoulder muscles. It could also be used as a 'stage one' to warm up the shoulders before advancing to either the Main Shoulder Flossing or Advanced Shoulder Flossing Moves.

STEP 1

SHOULDER FLEXION

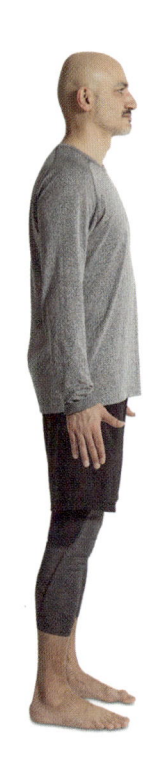

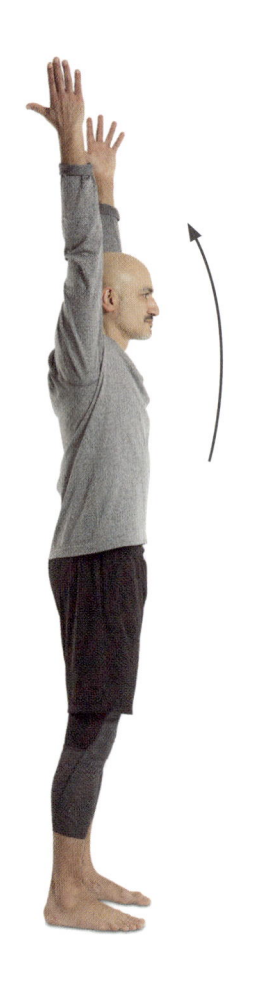

- Stand tall with your arms by your sides
- As you inhale, reach both arms up without hunching your shoulders.
- As you exhale, return your arms to your sides.
- Try to keep your shoulders down and relaxed as your raise up your arms.

REPS: Six.

STEP 2

SHOULDER EXTENSION

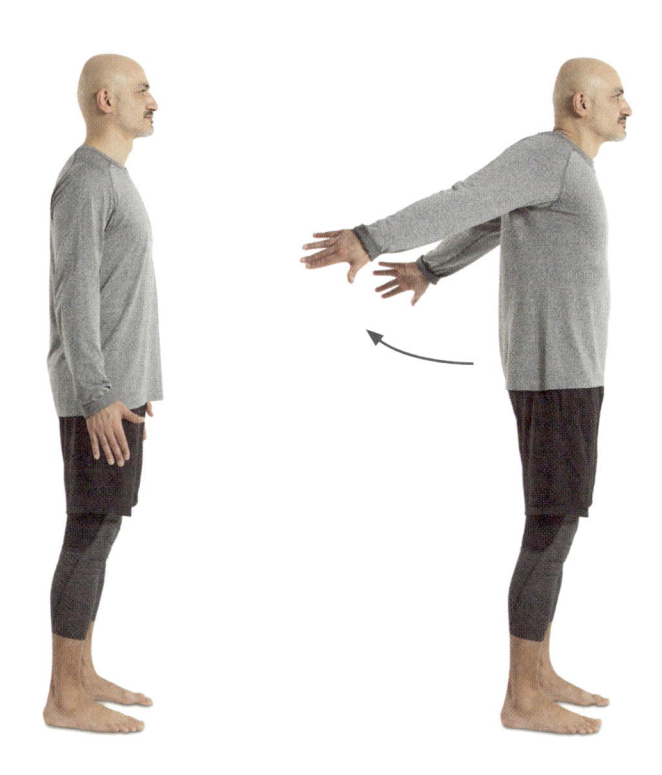

- Stand tall with your arms by your sides.
- As you inhale, reach both arms back without leaning forwards or hunching your shoulders.
- As you exhale, return your arms to your sides.
- Repeat, raising your arms a little higher each time.

REPS: Six.

MOVE 6: Gentle Shoulder Flossing

STEP 3

GENTLE BACK SCRATCHING

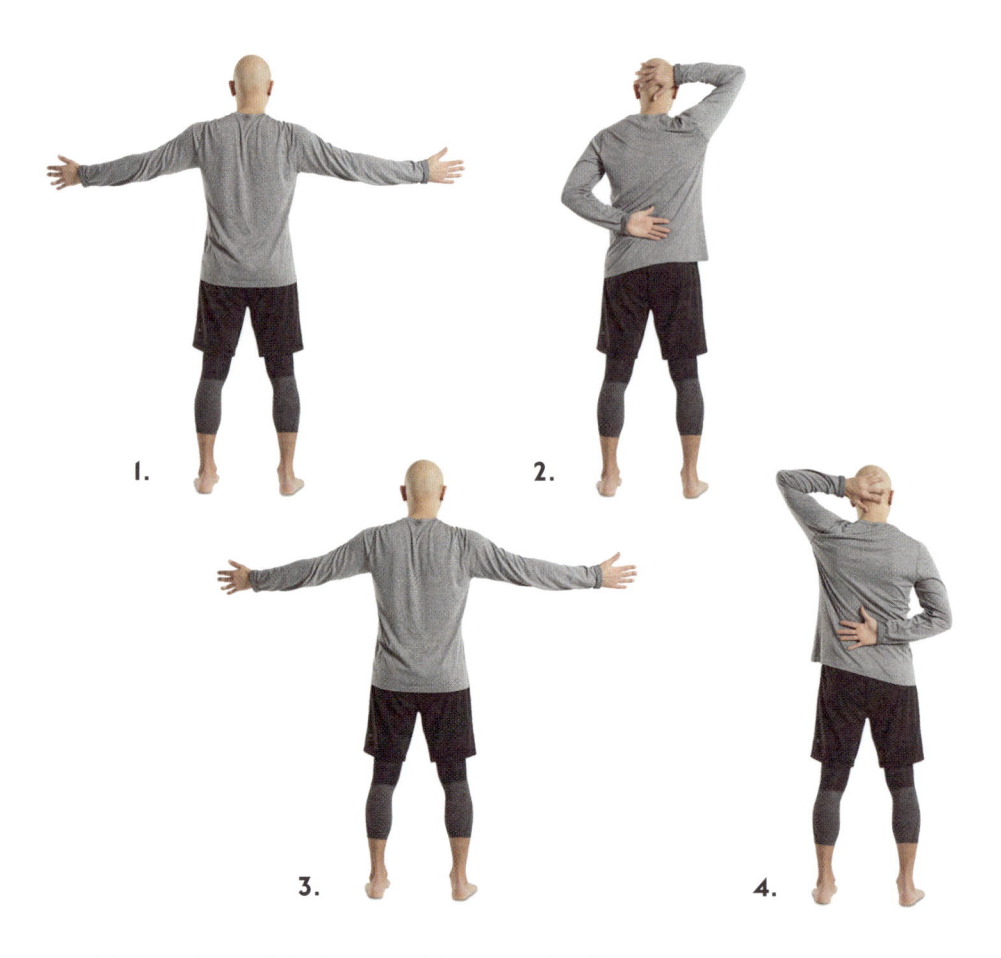

1.

2.

3.

4.

- Inhale and stretch both arms wide out to the sides.
- Exhale, place your right hand behind your head and your left hand on your lower back, palm facing outwards.
- Inhale and stretch both arms wide.
- Exhale, place your left hand behind your head and your right hand on your lower back.
- Repeat, inhaling to take the arms wide and exhaling as you bring your hands to the body.

REPS: Four on each side.

PLAY: Try leaving a gap by hovering your hands just away from your body.

STEP 4

ELBOW CIRCLING

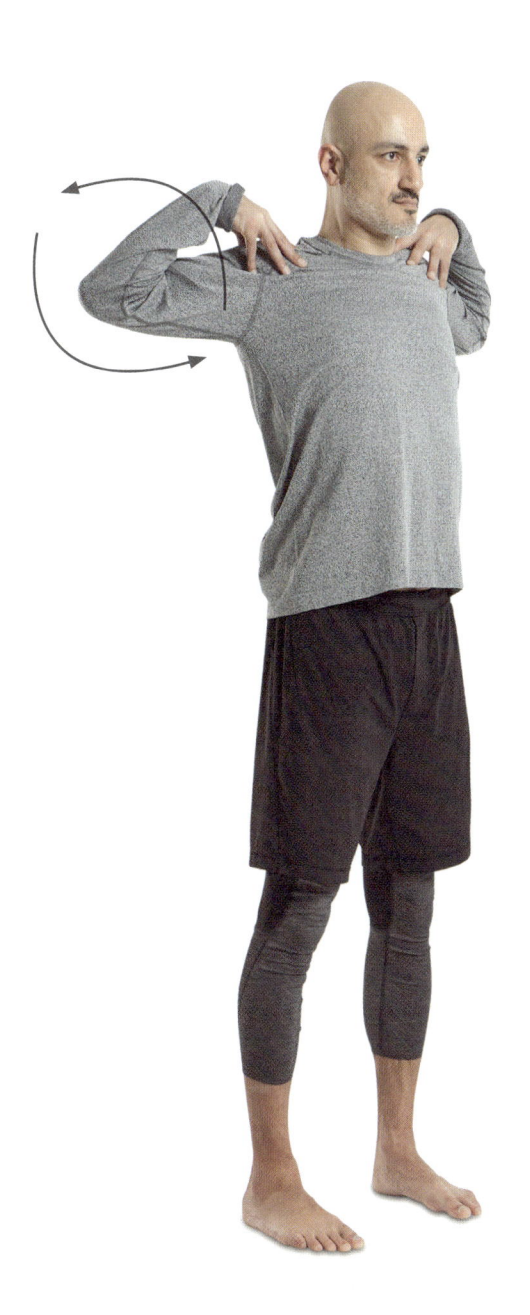

- Place your fingertips lightly on your shoulders.
- Circle both elbows at the same time.
- Breathe in and out slowly through the nose.

REPS: 10 (five clockwise and five anticlockwise).

PLAY: Switch to a swimming action by rotating first the right elbow forwards and then the left.

TIP: Do Elbow Circles at your desk to release shoulder tension.

MOVE 6: Gentle Shoulder Flossing

STEP 5

RELAXED SIDE STRETCH

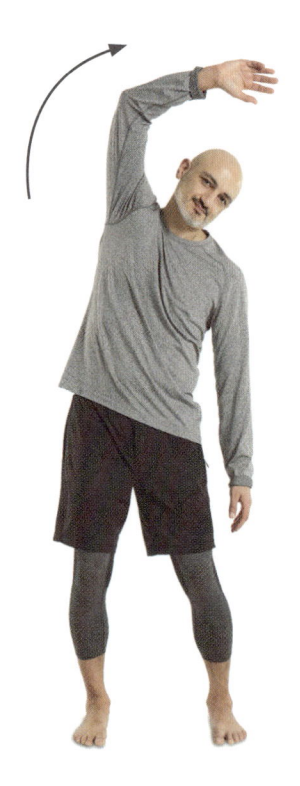

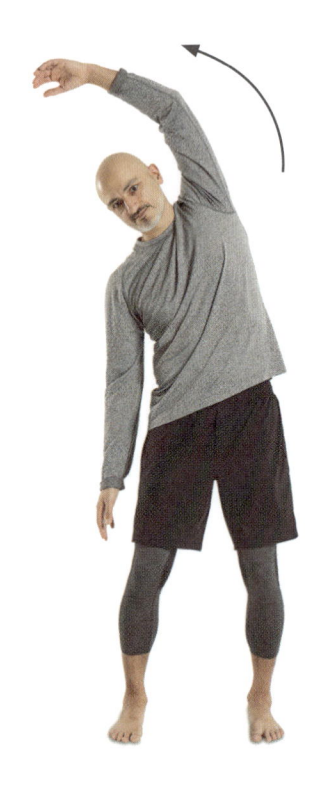

- Exhale and sweep your right arm up but keep it slightly bent.
- Lean to your left side.
- Inhale and return to the start position.
- Exhale, sweep your left arm up and lean to the right.
- Continue to move slowly and smoothly from side to side, inhaling to the centre and exhaling as you bend to the sides.

REPS: Four on each side.

STEP 6

RELAXED ROTATION

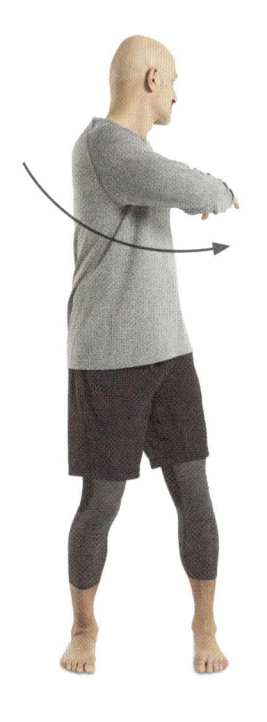

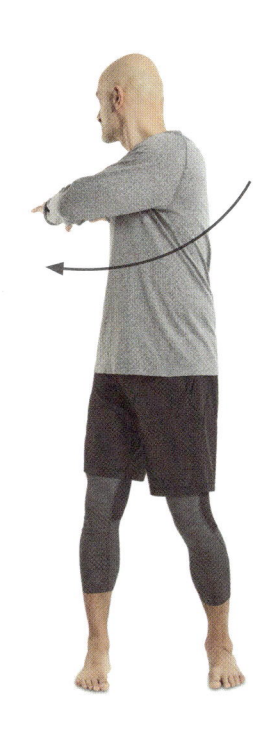

- Bend your knees and relax your arms by your sides. Or experiment by gradually raising the level of your arms to chest height and back down again while rotating.
- Begin to rotate your body from side to side.
- Allow your relaxed arms to spin with your body.
- Breathe in and out slowly through the nose.

REPS: Rotate for 20–30 seconds.

MOVE 6: Gentle Shoulder Flossing

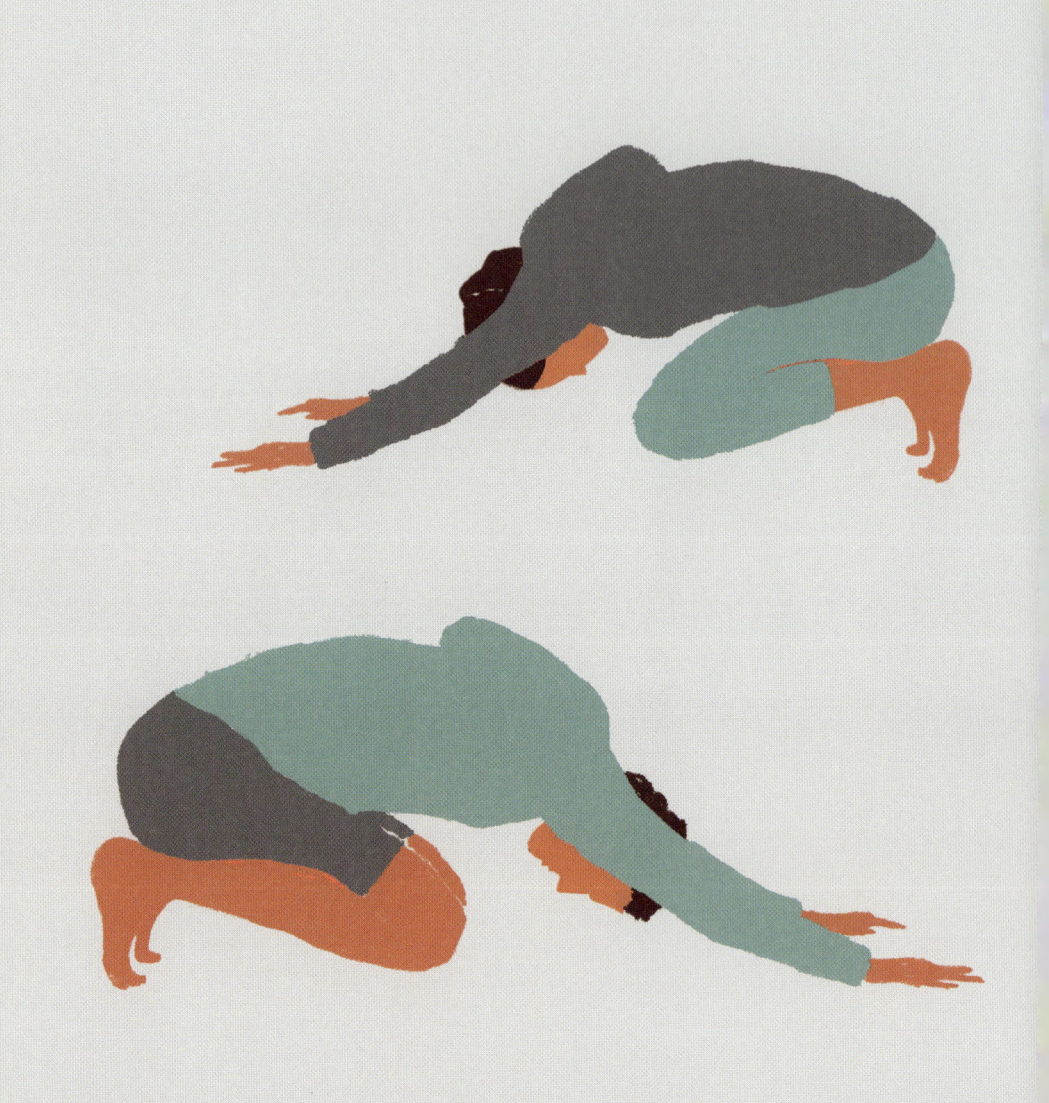

ADVANCED MOVES

If you are itching to lift the hips higher, rotate the torso deeper or sample a Seal, Inchworm or Scorpion then you've arrived at the right place.

Maybe you are already supple from doing martial arts, perfecting your squat form in the weights room, or flipping the Dog in yoga. Perhaps you've spent time practising the basic Moves and are primed for the next level.

These sequences are tougher versions of the six Main Moves, but what exactly does 'Advanced' mean? It's a good question, because flexibility is highly individual; what might seem like an impossible pretzel-like move to one person will be effortless for another.

The ways in which we've pushed the Moves up a notch for this section vary. The Advanced element might show up in the form of stronger back extension, such as the high Cobra performed in Advanced Cat Play, or complex shoulder acrobatics in Advanced Shoulder Flossing.

The Advanced Unstick the Hips and Hamstring Releasing Moves look much more like yoga than their Main and Gentle counterparts, as we tuck into deeper hip stretches and hairpin forward bends. However, it's not all about being bendy. Strength makes a few guest appearances, with planks or tricky balancing techniques scattered throughout.

With the Advanced label, though, comes a warning: for all movement that goes beyond our everyday range of motion, it's vital to watch the vulnerable areas of the body, especially the knees and lower back.

Knees are designed to bend back and forth like a hinge, not twist or rotate, so don't slide your front foot up too high in Pigeon Dips (Unstick the Hips), and if you feel any lower back discomfort in Seal (Cat Play), minimise the extension by lowering the upper body.

If you decide that these Moves are one step too far out of your comfort zone, please continue to play with the Main sequences. Or pick and mix Moves from the Main, Gentle and Advanced sections to create something tailor-made.

Ready for the challenge?

MOVE 1
ADVANCED BACK MOBILITY

Give your back a little love with this massaging, rolling, wrapping routine designed to assess which back muscles glide smoothly and which feel 'stuck' and in need of movement medicine. The supine (lying face up) position makes this a fantastic 'checking in' sequence suitable for even the bendiest yoga bunny, and a good 'stage one' to use as a warm-up for the other five Moves.

Things get a little more interesting in this version of the Back Mobility Move. It borrows the same techniques, designed to assess back movement, but mixes in leg wrapping, balancing and even a few crunches to earn the 'Advanced' tag.

Rising on to the tiptoes in Bridge gives us the luxury of more time and space to roll the back gradually down to the floor. The idea is to focus on laying the spine down in sections – almost vertebra by vertebra – to gain a deeper connection to the spine and release any tighter spots.

If you can't straighten the leg in the toe-tapping Advanced Thoracic Releaser exercise don't worry. Just keep it slightly bent, but try to glue both shoulders to the floor as you sweep the leg across the body.

As with all the Move techniques, work slowly and consciously, and synchronise the movement with the breathing. This usually means inhaling in the start position and exhaling as you slide into the movement.

Experiment with the leg wrapping shown in the final two techniques to see if it suits your back. By hooking one leg over the other we lock down the lower body to focus on upper body movement. If this causes any strain in your lower back, unwrap and stack one leg on top of the other.

Linking all six Moves together? Do this sequence first. However, if anything feels too much, too soon, flick back to the basic Back Mobility Move as your starting point.

STEP 1

ROLL AND BALANCE

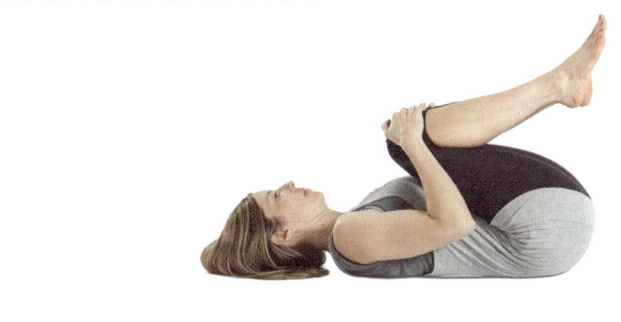

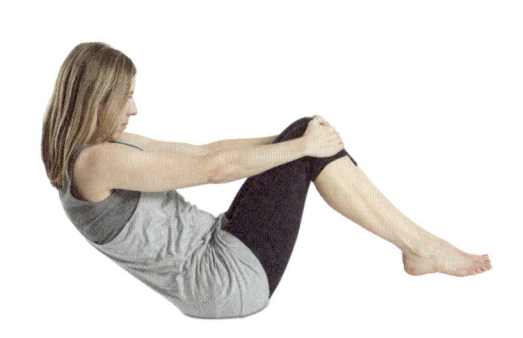

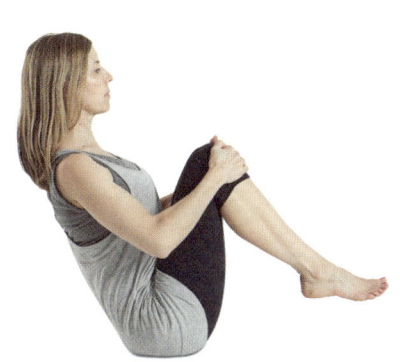

- Hug both legs tightly into your body
- Raise your head towards your knees to tuck into a ball.
- Rock up to sitting. Lift your chest and balance for a second or two.
- Tuck in your chin, round your back and roll back to the floor.
- Continue to roll up, balance and roll back to complete the reps.

REPS: Four.

PLAY: Engage the core as you balance to slow the roll-down part.

MOVE 1: Advanced Back Mobility

STEP 2

TIPTOE BRIDGES

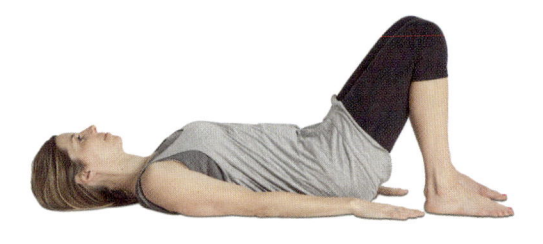

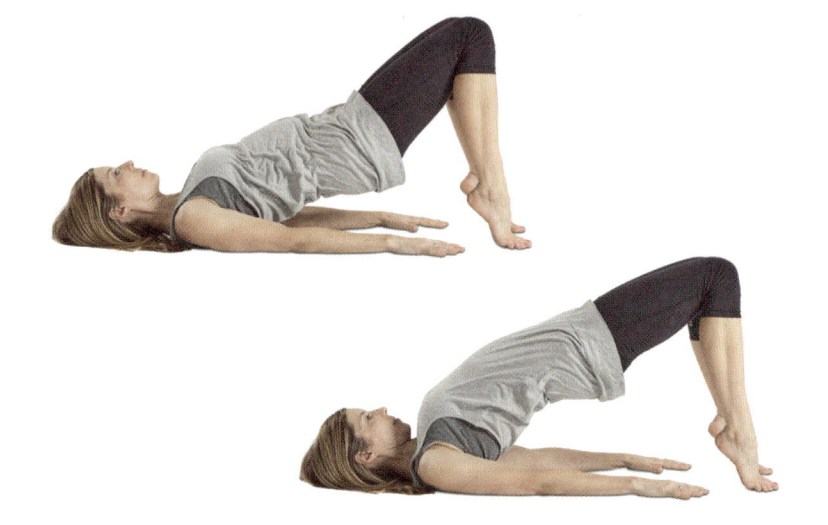

- Bend both legs and place your feet on the floor, hip-width apart.
- Place your arms by your side, palms facing down.
- Press your lower back into the floor.
- Inhale and peel your hips off the floor, then your mid-back, then your shoulder blades until you are in the Bridge position.
- Rise on to your tiptoes in Bridge and stay on your tiptoes as you exhale and lay your shoulder blades, mid-back and hips back on to the floor.
- Lower your heels as your hips touch down.
- Complete the reps, inhaling to peel the spine up, exhaling to lay it down..

REPS: Five.

PLAY: Raise your arms up above your head as you rise into Bridge. Return them slowly to your sides as you lower to the floor.

STEP 3

HUG AND CRUNCH

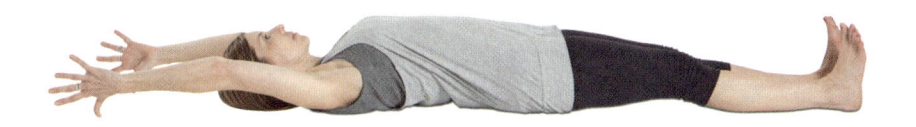

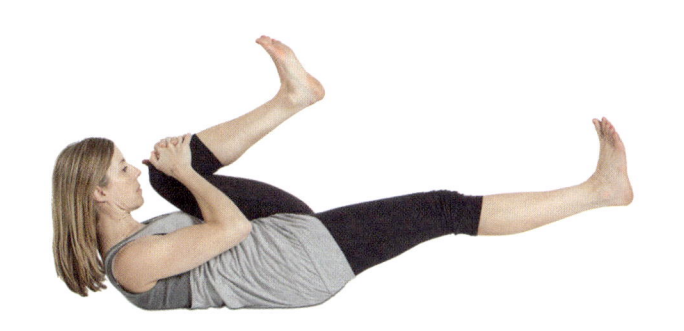

- Stretch your legs out straight with your toes pointing up.
- Place your arms by your sides, palms facing down.
- Inhale and sweep both arms above your head.
- Hug your right leg into your body and lift your head up, exhaling and bringing your nose towards your knee. Hold for a second.
- Lower down, then inhale and sweep both arms above your head.
- Hug your left leg into your body and lift your head, exhaling and bringing your nose towards your knee. Hold for a second.
- Continue switching from leg to leg. Inhale to sweep the arms up and exhale to crunch.

REPS: Six on each side.

STEP 4

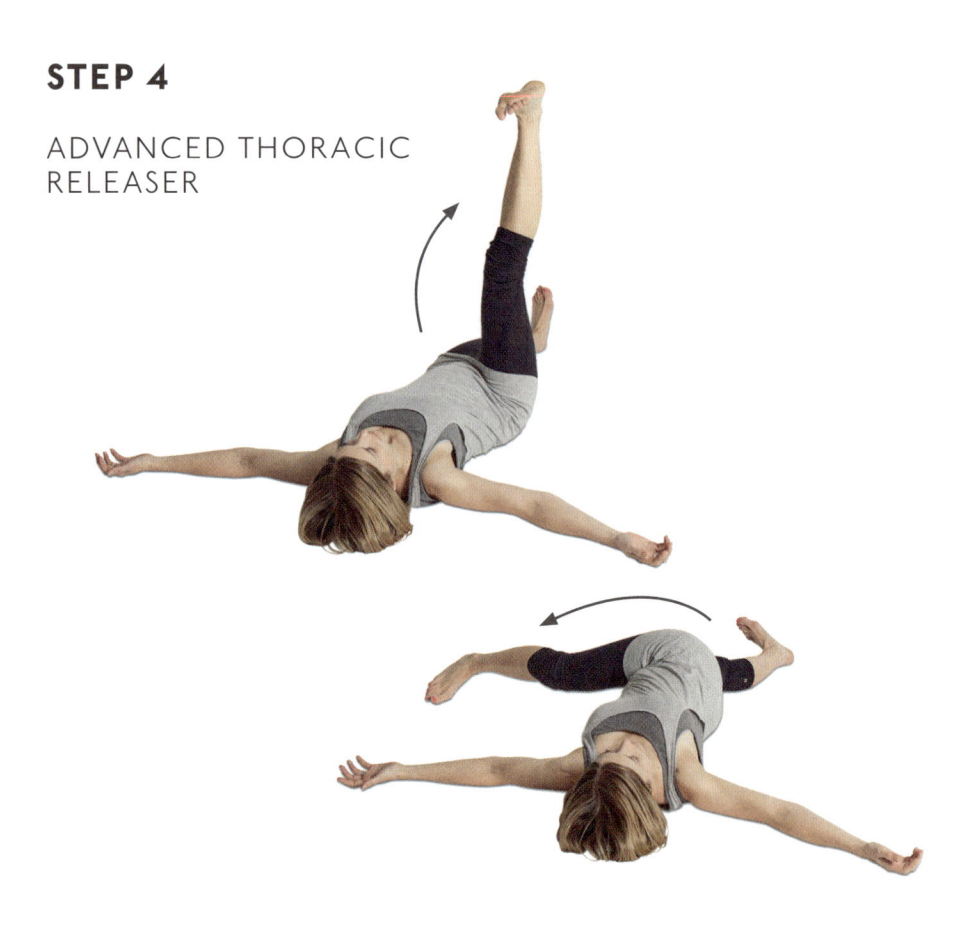

ADVANCED THORACIC RELEASER

- Hug your right knee in and press your lower back slightly to the floor.
- Stretch your arms out on the floor at shoulder height, palms facing up.
- Straighten your right leg up towards the ceiling so it forms a 90-degree angle with your body (bend the leg a little if required).
- Inhale here. As you exhale, swing your straight leg across your body and tap your toes to the floor on the left of your body.
- Inhale to return the leg to the centre.
- Keep both shoulders stuck to the floor throughout.
- Complete the reps, then switch legs.

REPS: Five on each side.

STEP 5

ADVANCED BOOK PAGES

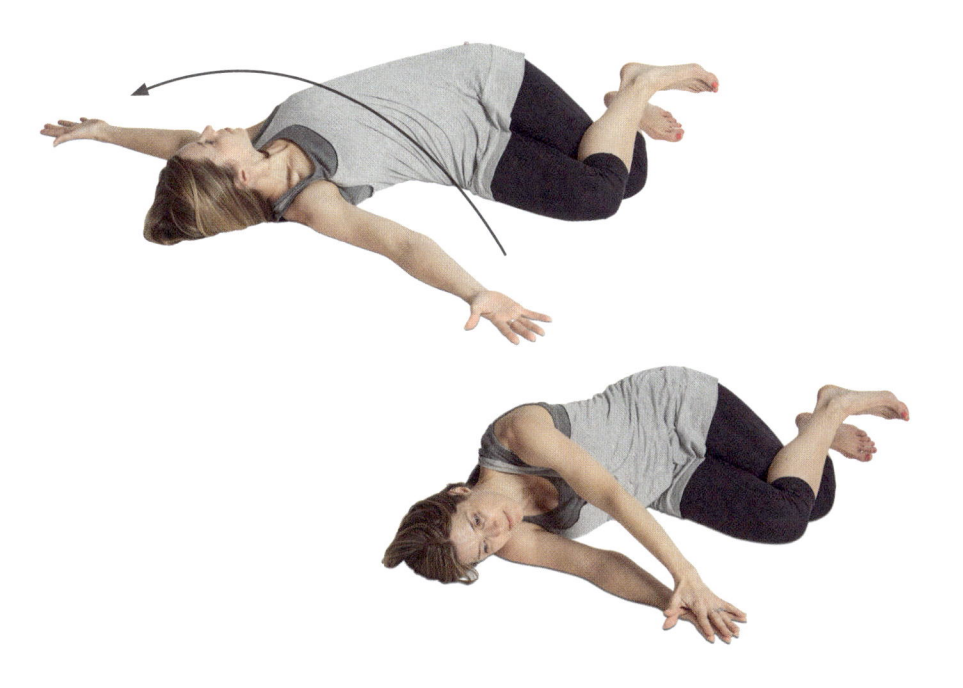

- Bend both legs and position your feet a little wider than hip-width apart.
- Stretch your arms out on the floor at shoulder height, palms facing up.
- Lower both legs to the right side without moving your feet.
- Slide your right leg out and rest your right ankle on top of your left thigh.
- Inhale in this position. As you exhale, lift your left arm up and roll on to your right side, placing both palms together.
- Inhale to open the arms wide again.
- Complete the reps, then switch sides by rolling on to your left side and resting your left ankle on top of your right thigh. Sweep your right arm over and back.

REPS: Four on each side.

STEP 6

ADVANCED SHOULDER CLOCKS

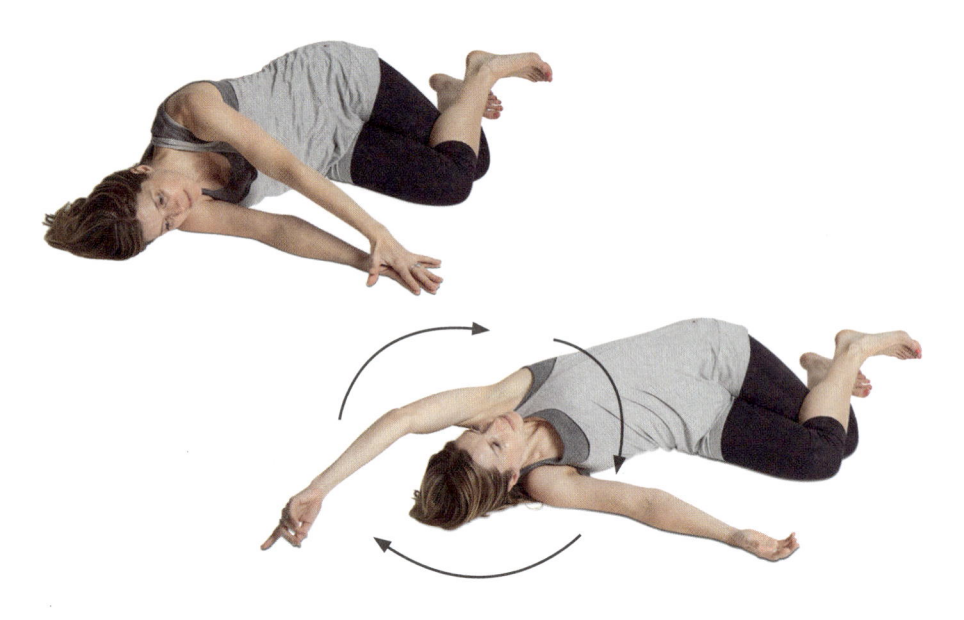

- Return to the Advanced Book Pages start position with your right leg hooked on top of your left thigh.
- Roll on to your right side and place your palms together.
- Trace a large circular movement with your left arm by circling it overhead and out to the left.
- Trace three circles in a clockwise direction and three anticlockwise.
- Keep the breath flowing as you circle.
- Complete the reps and switch sides by rolling on to your left side and resting your left ankle of top of your right thigh. Circle your right arm.

REPS: Six on each side.

TIP: Try to keep your fingertips on the floor as you trace the circles.

CHANGE IT UP

If you want it more gentle...
For a less-strenuous version of this Move, see page 86.

MOVE 2
ADVANCED CAT PLAY

Cats are joined by seals, scorpions, canines and cobras in this powerful, animal inspired flow. We fuse flexibility training with core control and strength work to concoct a challenging, playful sequence for the back, shoulders and beyond. The sequence ends with an invitation to explore in slow motion, so ease off the speed and substitute mechanical movement for mindful.

The idea is to transition smoothly through all the movements a healthy back loves. There is plenty of flexion and extension, but also rotation and side stretching, in order to target different back zones:

Sitting Cats loosens up the lower or lumber region.
Scorpions focuses on mobility for the mid-, or thoracic, back.
Shoulder Blade Taps and Shoulder Dips are a test of upper back and shoulder flexibility.

Our last sequence – Rolling – is not easy! It's a test of core conditioning, back flexibility, arm strength and (last but not least) patience. The knee bend in the squat creates a nice coiled spring effect, but don't rush it. It's tempting to spring from A to B – or squat to plank – quickly. Instead, slow down the technique to ripple the spine through a flexed position halfway before straightening out to plank. This demands excellent spinal mobility, core control and concentration.

As ever, the golden rules apply: never push beyond your natural movement boundaries, and move slowly. As with all the Moves, I have included suggestions for when to breathe in or out. This elevates these Moves away from purely mechanical exercises to a dance or flow, and also allows you time to move consciously and carefully.

STEP 1

SITTING CATS

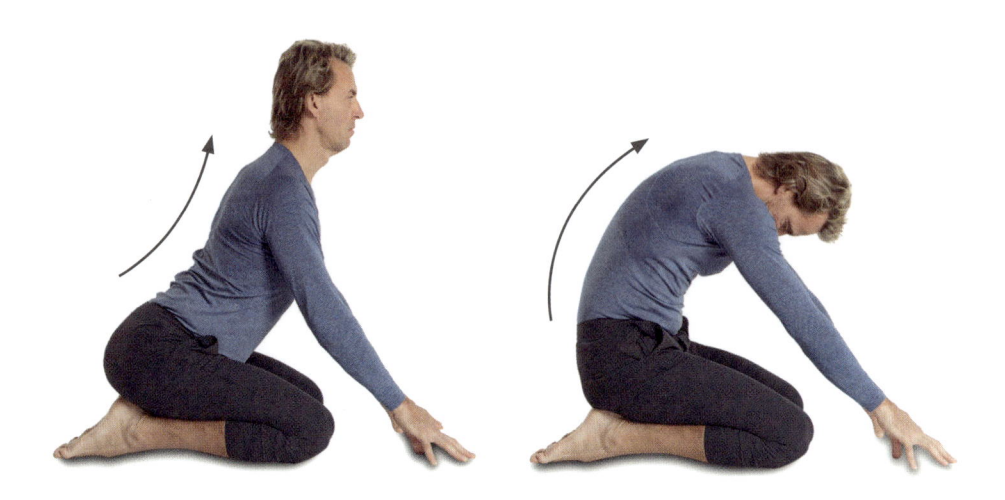

- Sit in a kneeling position.
- Walk your hands forwards along the floor until your arms are straight, and spread your fingers on the floor.
- As you inhale, arch or extend your back and look forwards.
- As you exhale, round or flex your back, tuck in your chin and lean away from your fingertips.
- Continue to extend and flex your spine to complete the reps, synchronising the movement with your breathing.

REPS: Six.

STEP 2

SHOULDER DIPS

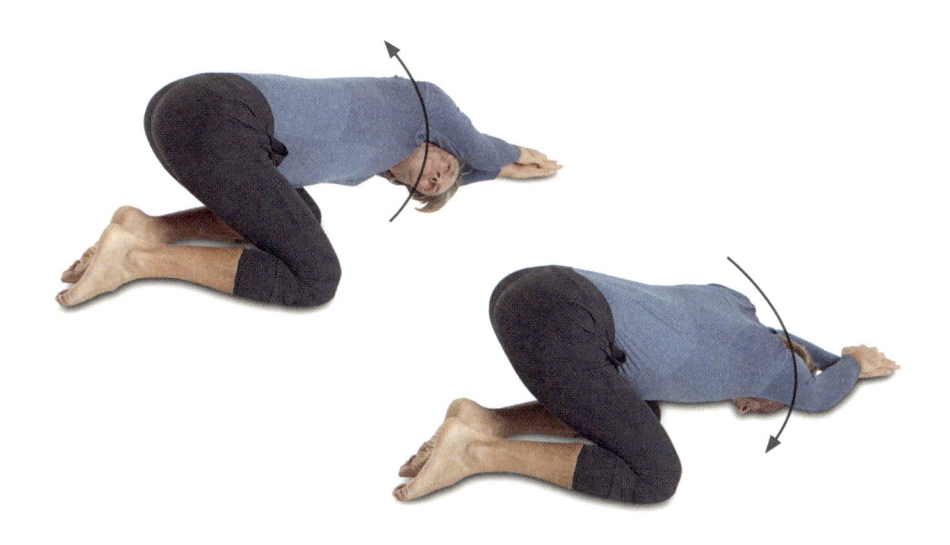

- Stay kneeling but lower your forehead to the floor and stretch your arms overhead on the floor, walking your fingertips as far as they'll go.
- Walk both hands around to the left.
- Place your right hand on top of your left and interlink the fingers around your left hand.
- Imagine both hands are stuck to the floor, then lean away from them to feel a deep side stretch.
- Now lift and lower your right shoulder by dropping it up and down towards the floor to complete the reps.
- Inhale as you lift the shoulder and exhale to drop it down.
- Walk both hands round to the right side and repeat.

REPS: Five on each side.

MOVE 2: Advanced Cat Play

STEP 3

SHOULDER BLADE TAPS

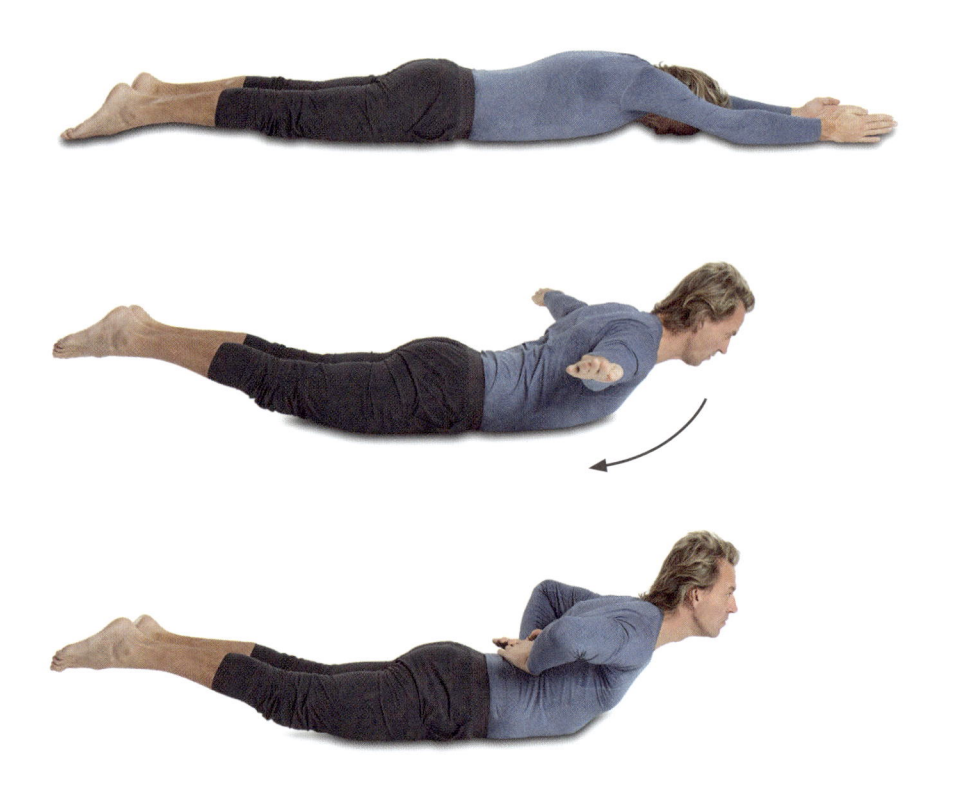

- Lie on your front with your forehead on the floor.
- Stretch your arms above your head on the floor, palms facing down.
- Inhale and lift your whole body off the floor. Sweep both arms behind your back so that your thumbs touch your shoulder blades on the upper back.
- Exhale and return to your start position by sweeping your arms back above your head and lowering the body to the floor.

REPS: Four.

STEP 4

SEAL FLOW

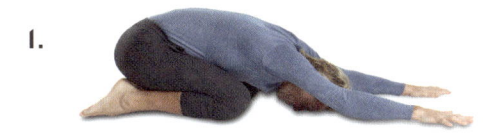

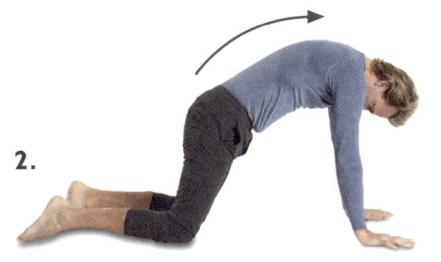

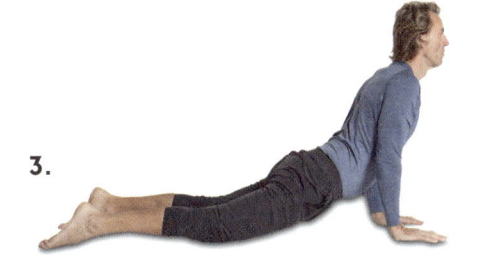

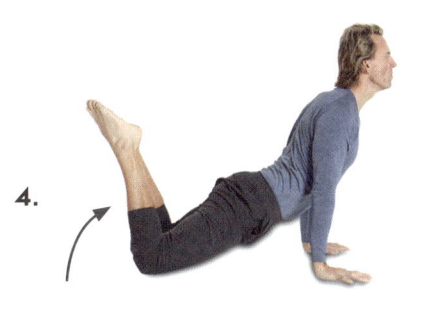

1.

2.

3.

4.

- Return to kneeling with your forehead on the floor and arms stretched above your head.
- Spread your fingers and press your palms into the floor.
- Rise up to the all-fours Cat position with your back rounded and chin tucked in.
- Keep moving forwards until your hips drop down, then lower the rest of your body slowly to the floor.
- Simultaneously press into your hands and lift your upper body while bending your legs and bringing your feet towards your buttocks. This is Seal. Squeeze your buttocks in the leg-lifting part to protect the back.
- To reverse, lower your feet, lift back into Cat and sit back on your heels.
- Continue. Keep your breath flowing in and out as you move.

REPS: Four.

MOVE 2: Advanced Cat Play

STEP 5

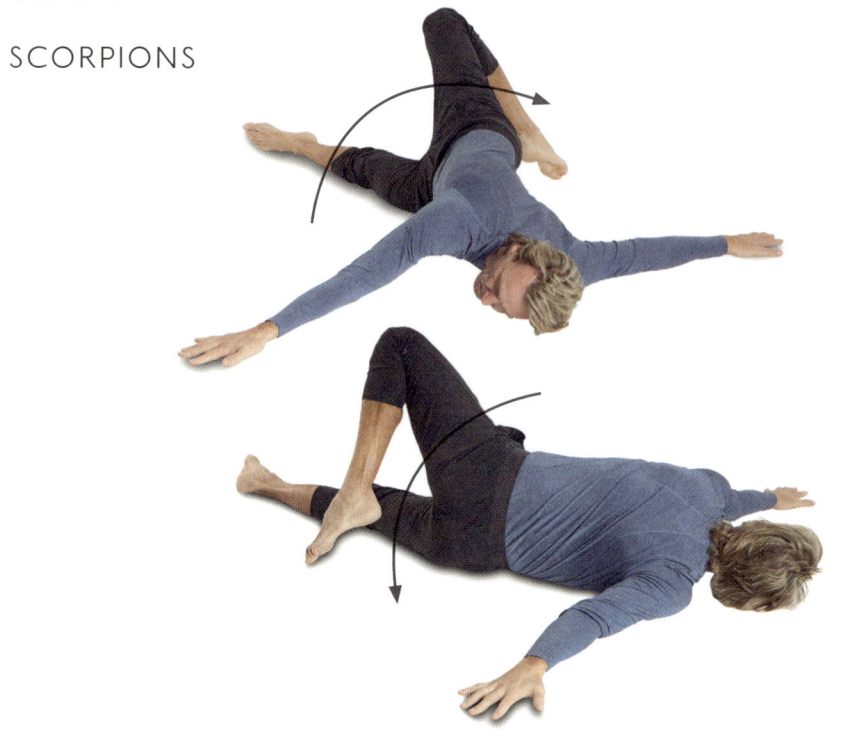

SCORPIONS

- Lie on your front with your forehead on the floor. Stretch your arms out on the floor at shoulder height, palms facing down.
- Bend your left leg, inhale and lift your knee off the floor.
- Swing your left leg across to your right side. The left toes might touch the floor but don't force this movement if not.
- Return to the start position.
- Bend your right leg, inhale and lift your knee off the floor.
- Swing your right leg across to your right side.
- Return to the start position.
- Keep your breathing flowing in and out as you move.

REPS: Four on each side.

STEP 6

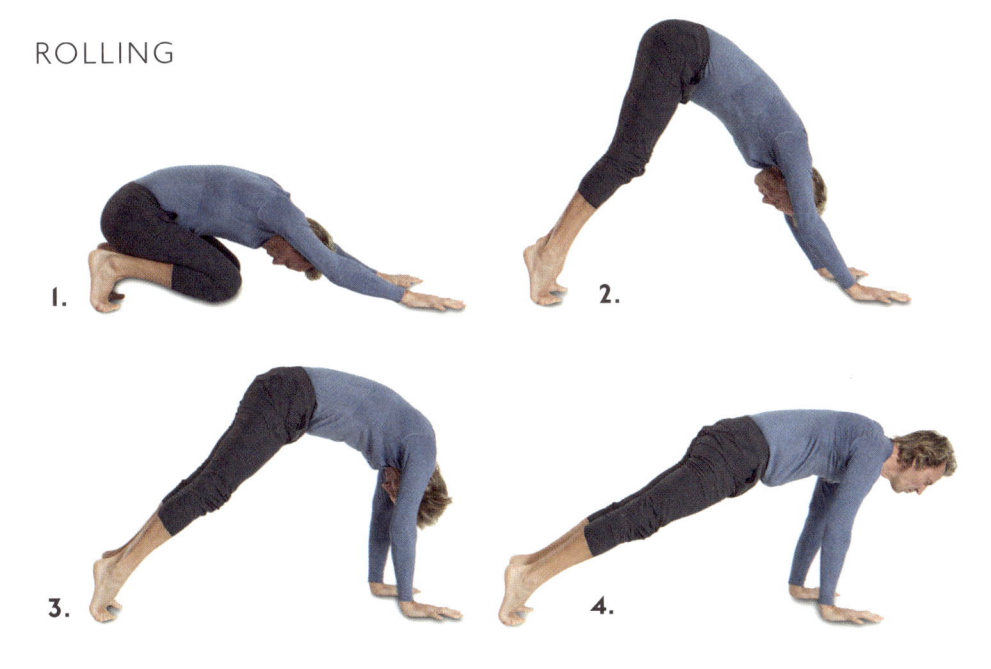

ROLLING

1.
2.
3.
4.

- Come to all fours and tuck your toes under.
- Without moving your hands, lift your knees off the floor and squat back towards your heels.
- Begin to straighten your legs, rise high on to your tiptoes, lift your hips and flex your back to form a high Cat position.
- Continue to move forwards, gradually lowering the hips until the body straightens out into a plank position with heels, hips and head in line.
- Reverse the movement. Lift your hips, flex your back and rise high on to your tiptoes. Keep moving backwards until you are squatting back on your heels.
- Continue to roll from squat to plank slowly and with control.
- Keep the breath flowing in and out as you move.

REPS: Four.

TIP: Try rolling in slow motion.

MOVE 2: Advanced Cat Play

MOVE 3
ADVANCED UNSTICK THE HIPS

Good hip mobility is crucial for boosting athletic power, preventing lower back pain and offsetting the muscle-shortening impact of hours spent sitting. Here's a dynamic sequence to improve hip movement inspired by techniques from the yoga studio as well as the weights room. Don't expect to fold into a full lotus. Do expect to a) have fun and b) own hips that move well.

What do you get if you mix squat mobility drills from the gym with flow yoga and add a pinch of animal inspired moves? Something like this hip movement cocktail!

This Move is for anyone who already has above-average hip mobility and wants an active, challenging routine to advance this range of motion.

We start with Hip Circling but with straight legs to also warm up the hamstrings, then move on to Sweep and Reach, which incorporates the broad muscles of the back and sides that play a role in keeping the hips supple.

Squat Folds offers a little more hamstring stretching and 90 Drop and Lift gives us a chance to stretch the hips, combined with a little shoulder strengthening.

Pigeon Dips is a variation of yoga's famous deep glute-stretching pose, Pigeon, but take care of your knee when you set it up. Slide the foot too high to increase the knee angle and you risk placing undue pressure on a joint that is essentially a hinge and doesn't like to be over-rotated.

Another yoga pose – one of the seated spinal twists – completes the set. This is a dynamic, looser version of the pose that's designed to allow the shoulders to rotate to face forwards and then slide to the sides. So, don't hug the front leg too tightly to your torso or you'll prevent the upper body from moving freely.

Enjoy playing with some next-level movements for the hips, hamstrings, back and beyond.

STEP 1

HIP CIRCLING

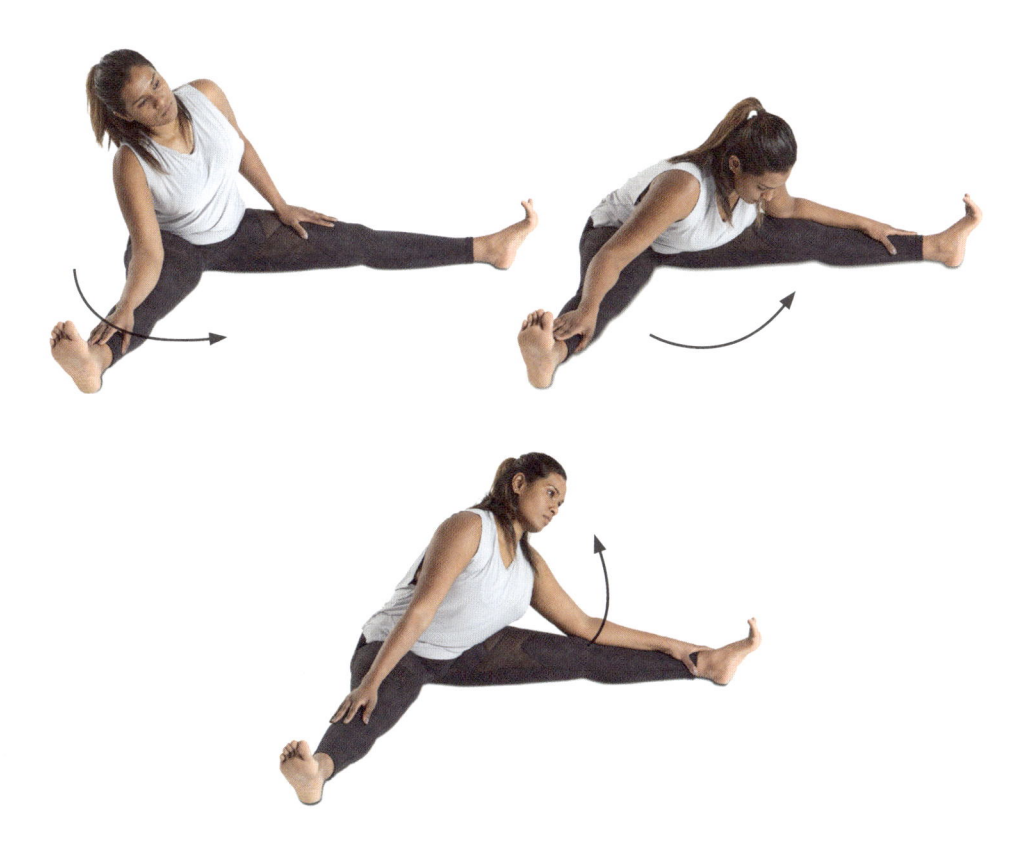

- Sit tall with your legs straight and spread wide. Point your toes up.
- Place your hands on your thighs.
- Slowly circle your upper body, leaning forwards, to the sides and back.
- Continue, breathing in and out as you move.

REPS: Circle for 10–20 seconds.

TIP: Sit cross-legged if tight hamstrings are restricting the movement.

STEP 2

SWEEP AND REACH

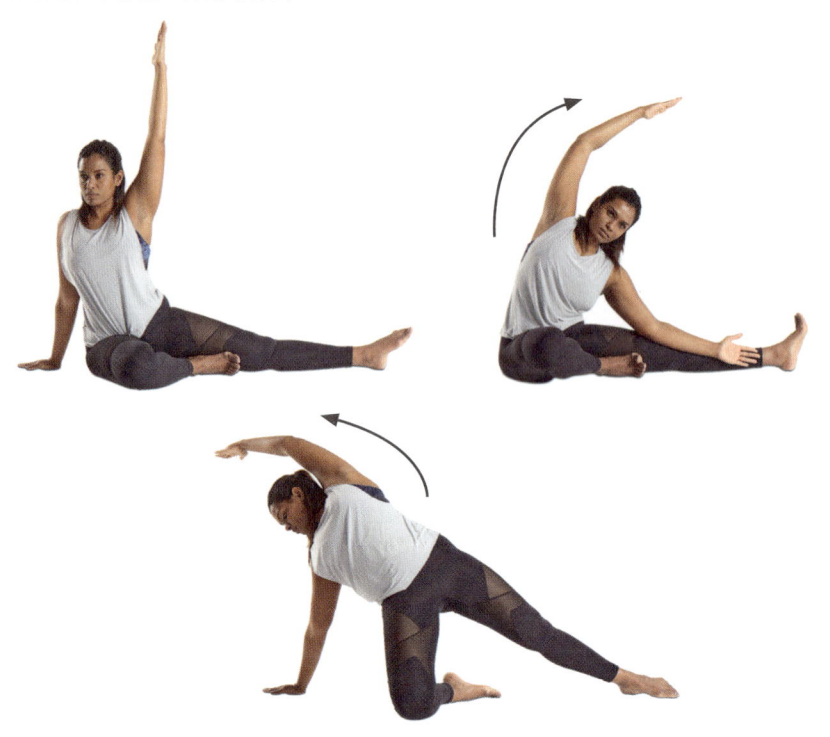

- Stay sitting with wide legs.
- Bend your right leg and place the sole of the right foot on the inside of your left thigh. Sit tall. Place your right hand on the floor behind you.
- Inhale, press into the right hand, lift your hips high and sweep your left arm over by your head.
- Lower to your start position.
- Reach your right arm up and lean over your straight leg.
- Continue moving between the two positions, inhaling to lift your hips and exhaling to lean over your leg.
- Complete the reps and switch sides by bending your left leg and placing your left hand behind your back.

REPS: Four on each side.

STEP 3

SQUAT FOLDS

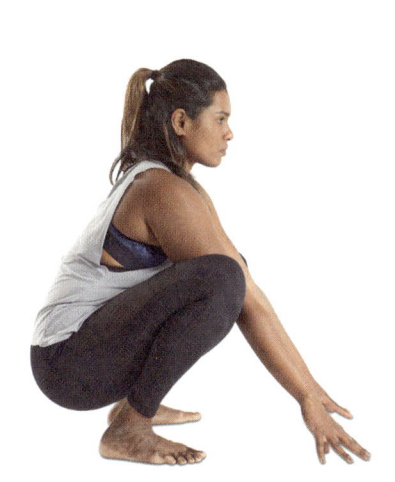

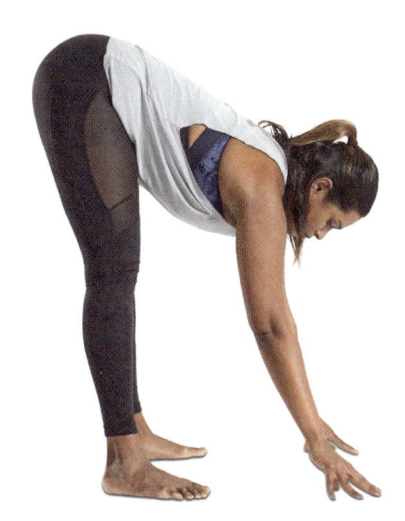

- Perform a low squat with your feet a bit wider than hip-width apart, toes turned slightly outwards, hips dropped low and both fingertips on the floor.
- Exhale, straighten your legs and lower your head to fold forwards.
- Inhale, raise your upper body, bend your legs and return to the squat.
- Alternate between the two positions, keeping your fingertips on the floor throughout.

REPS: Four.

PLAY: If your heels don't reach the floor in the squat think about dropping them a touch lower on each rep.

MOVE 3: Advanced Unstick the Hips

STEP 4

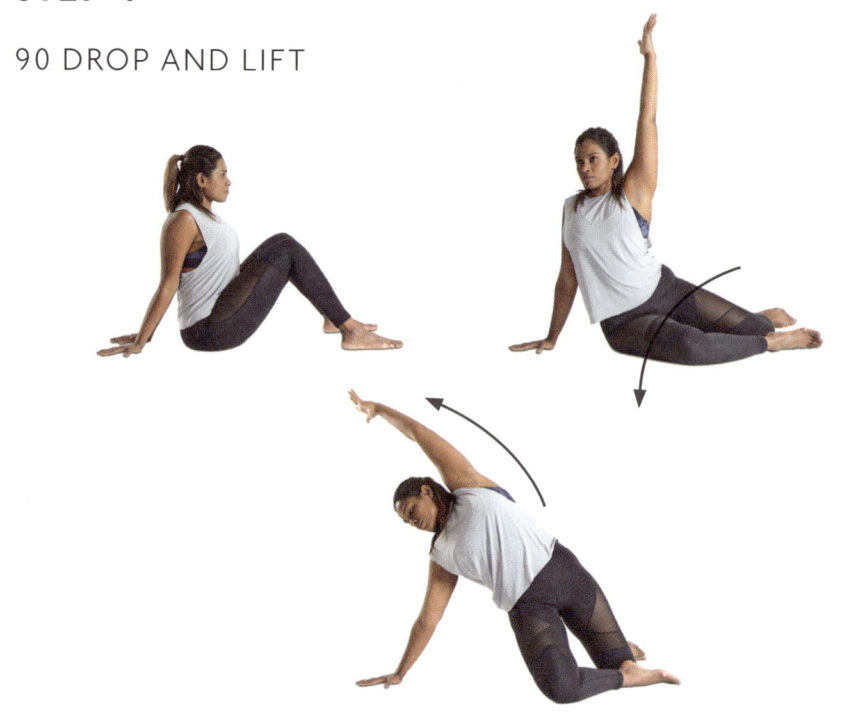

90 DROP AND LIFT

- Sit on the floor with your legs bent into a 90-degree position and your feet a bit wider than hip-width apart.
- Lean back, rest your hands on the floor and lift your chest.
- Without moving your feet drop both knees to the floor on the right side.
- Lean on your right hand, lift your hips high and reach your left arm over by your head.
- Lower your arm and then sit back down on the floor.
- Drop both knees to the floor on the left side.
- Lean on your left hand, lift your hips high and reach your right arm over by your head
- Exhale to drop the knees to the side and inhale to lift the hips.

REPS: Three on each side.

STEP 5

PIGEON DIPS

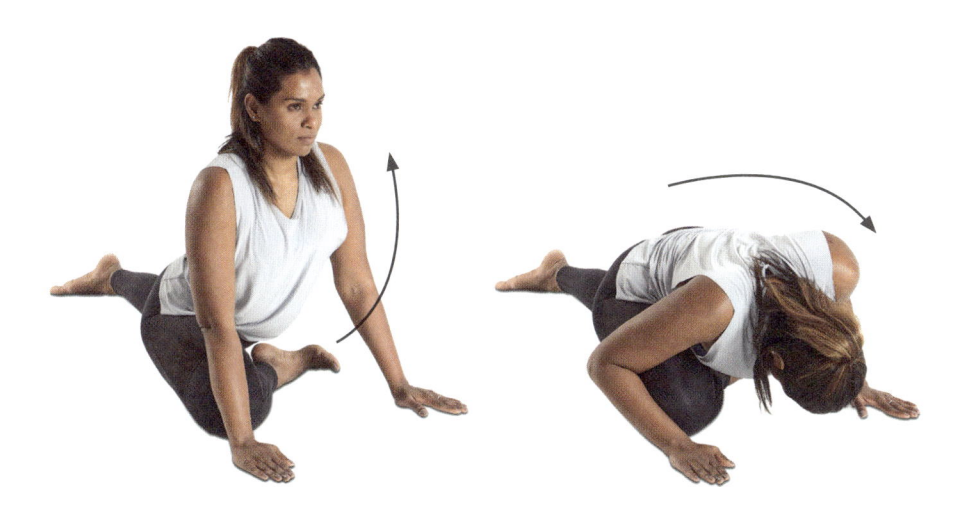

- Come to all fours with your hands under your shoulders.
- Slide your right knee behind your right wrist and wiggle your foot a little over to the left (but not so far that it stresses the knee).
- Straighten your left leg and slide it out behind you, in line with your left hip.
- Inhale, straighten your arms and lift your chest.
- As you exhale, bend both arms, keeping your elbows tucked into your sides, and dip your upper body down to the floor.
- Inhale and lift your chest.
- Complete the reps, then switch sides.

REPS: Five on each side.

PLAY: Lightly tap your nose to the floor on each dip.

MOVE 3: Advanced Unstick the Hips

STEP 6

HUG AND TWIST

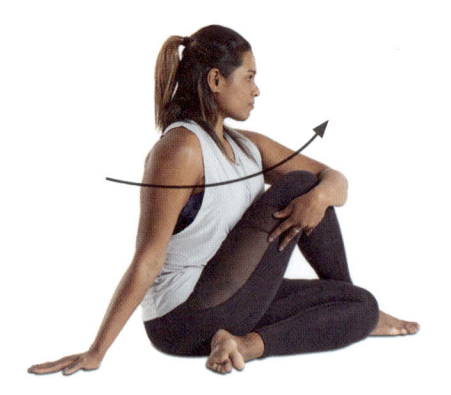

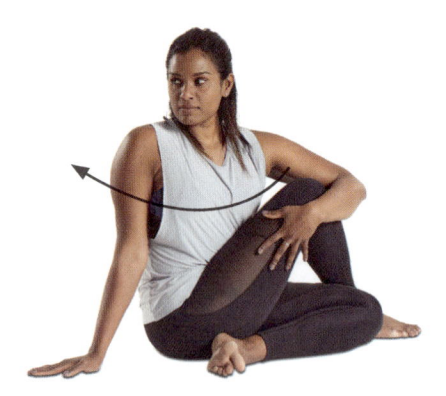

- Sit tall with your legs stretched out straight and toes pointing up.
- Step your right foot over your left thigh.
- Lean to the left, bend your left leg and tuck it in towards your hips.
- Sit tall, ensuring both buttocks are on the floor.
- Wrap your left arm around your right leg and hug.
- Place your right hand behind your back.
- Sit tall, exhale and turn your shoulders to the right
- Inhale and turn your shoulders to face front
- Continue, rotating the upper body to the right and back. Inhale to face front and exhale as you rotate.
- Complete the reps, then unravel and switch legs.

REPS: Four on each side.

CHANGE IT UP

If you want it more gentle...
For a less-strenuous version of this Move, see page 100.

MOVE 4
ADVANCED LUNGE FLOW

Harness your inner ninja with these stealthy moves for the hip flexors, hamstrings, quads and more. The goal is to hold a deep lunge to 'open' the hips and chest while we get busy releasing the upper body through lateral stretching and rotation. It's the perfect antidote to a 'closed' or flexed seated workplace position, and a great hip release for cyclists, hikers or runners.

We drop low to the ground with plenty of crawling, rocking and sliding with these ninja-style stealth moves. Our main anatomical point of focus is the iliopsoas or 'hip flexors' at the front of the hips but we'll also free up the quads, groin and hamstrings along the way. Women tend to find this type of deep hip movement easier than men, partly due to generally superior hamstring flexibility, and a wider pelvis, but rules are made to be broken! With dedicated practice the hip muscles will begin to respond with increased mobility.

This Move is ideal for hikers, runners and cyclists who already possess a good degree of flexibility, and anyone whose job requires them to sit for much of the day. The plan is to keep you fixed in the lunge while we play with additional upper-body movement, meaning that your hip flexors get a really long release. Pad your back knee with a foam yoga block or cushion, if necessary.

The usual Move rules apply: never force yourself into a position that feels rigid and locked (we want *more* movement, not less), and ease in and out of any movements slowly.

This last rule applies particularly to our final ninja technique, Side Lunging. Here, the knees are deeply flexed and, therefore, vulnerable to injury. Slide slowly and ensure your knee tracks in line with your toes. Having a bad knee day? Revert to the basic Lunge Flow Move by placing your hands on your thighs and keeping the soles of the feet on the floor as you glide from side to side.

> **Start with your right leg forwards and move through the entire flow, then repeat the sequence with the left foot in front.**

TIP: TRY PERFORMING THIS SEQUENCE IN SLOW MOTION.

STEP 1

SLIDING

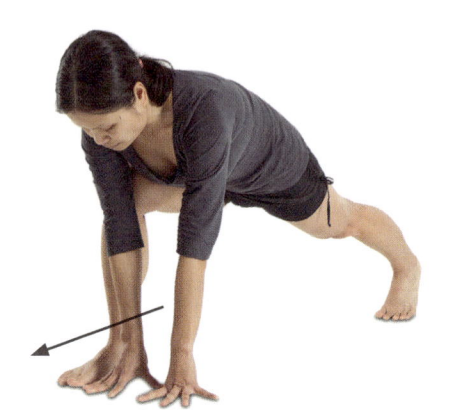

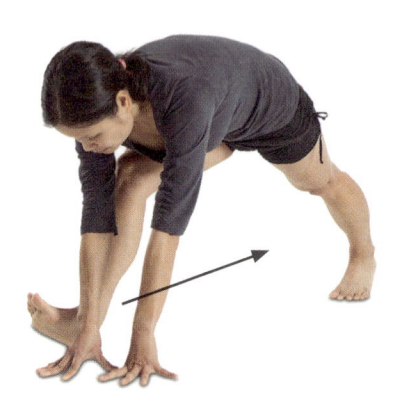

- From all fours, step your right foot up to the outside of your right hand.
- Roll on to the edge of your right foot and let your right knee drop out.
- As you inhale, drop your hips and sink lower into the lunge.
- As you exhale, move your hips back.
- Repeat to complete the reps, rocking forwards and backwards.
- If you want to lunge deeper, roll onto the edge of your right foot and let your right knee drop out.

REPS: Five.

STEP 2

ARM CIRCLING

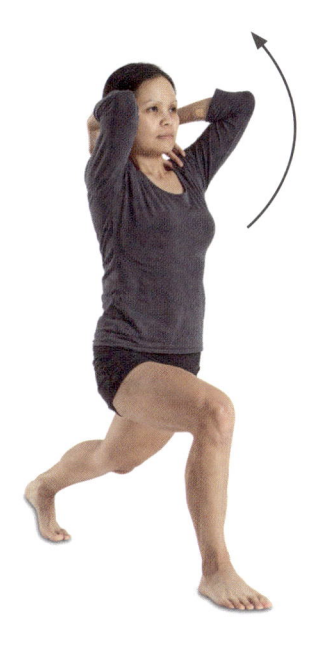

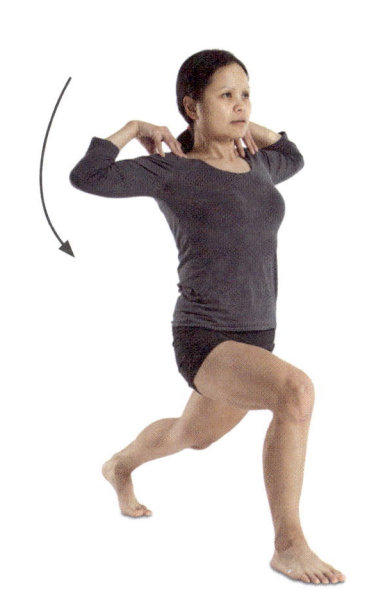

- Tuck your back toes under and lift your back knee off the floor to create a balancing lunge.
- Make slow circles with both arms.
- Inhale to sweep them up and exhale to bring them down.

REPS: Six.

PLAY: Try to make the roundest circles possible.

MOVE 4: Advanced Lunge Flow

STEP 3

ELBOW POINTING

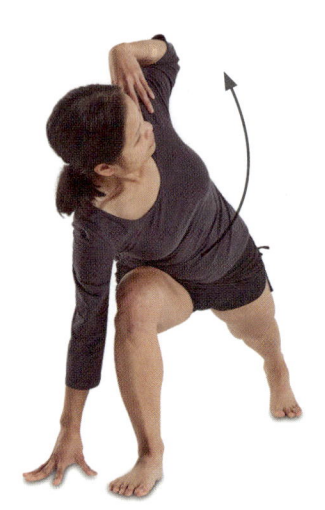

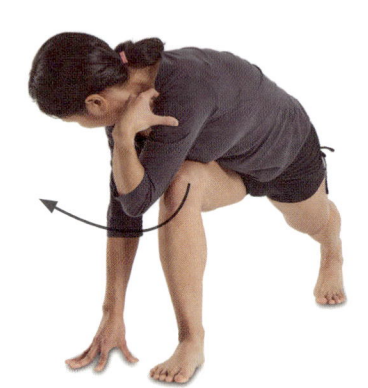

- Place your left hand on your left shoulder. Drop your right fingertips to rest on the floor on your right side.
- As you inhale, point the left elbow behind you.
- As you exhale, sweep the arm past your right leg and point the elbow down to the floor.
- Repeat, pointing the elbow back and down.

REPS: Five.

STEP 4

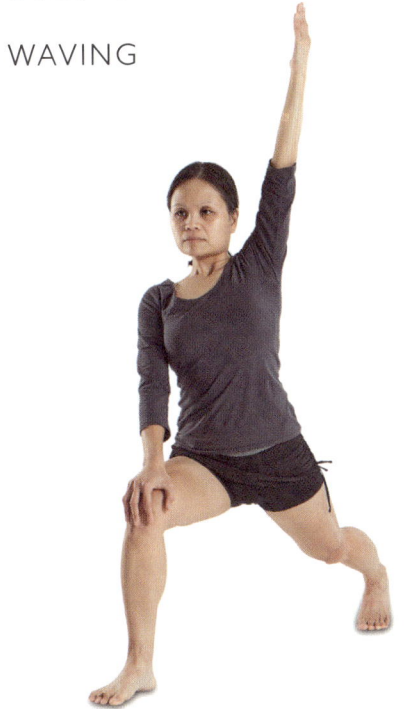

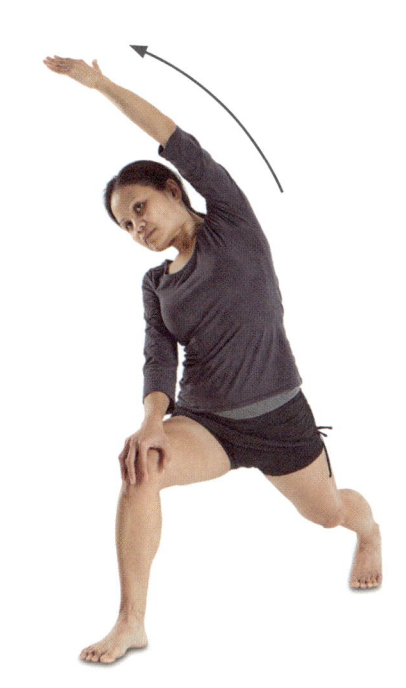

WAVING

- Place your hand on your knee.
- Reach your left arm up above your head. Inhale here.
- As you exhale, sweep your left arm over to the right.
- Repeat, inhaling to the centre and exhaling over.

REPS: Five.

PLAY: Try sweeping the arm across the body at chest height to create more torso rotation.

MOVE 4: Advanced Lunge Flow

STEP 5

LUNGE TWISTING

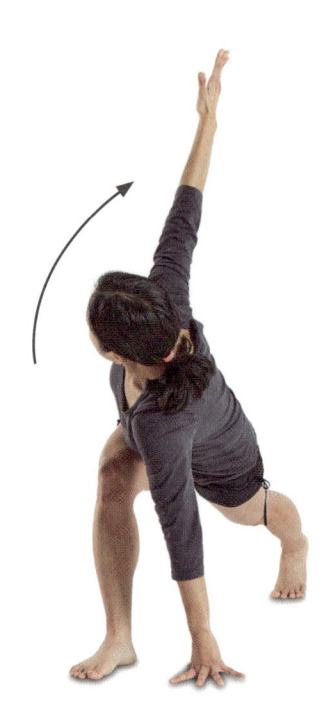

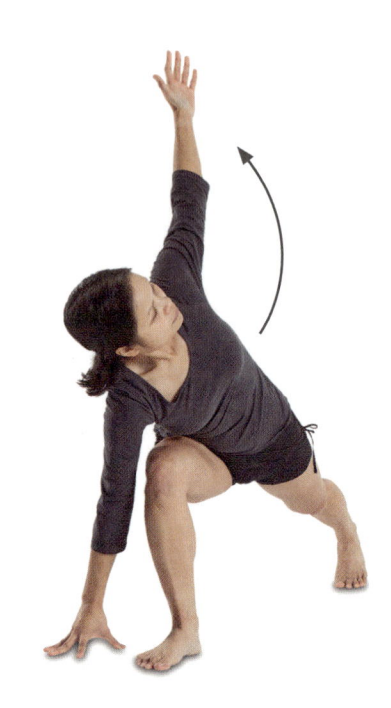

- Place one hand either side of your right front foot again.
- As you inhale, reach your right arm up. As you exhale, return it to the ground.
- As you inhale, reach your left arm up. As you exhale, return it to the ground.
- Continue, twisting slowly from side to side.

REPS: Four.

STEP 6

SIDE LUNGING

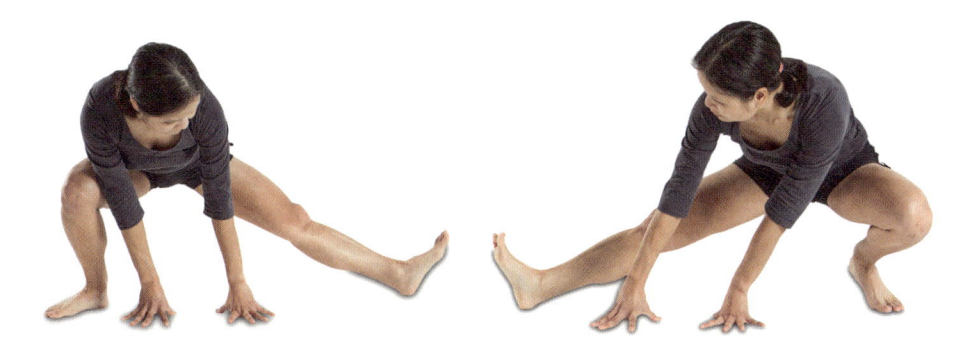

- Stand with your feet much wider than hip-width apart and turn your toes slightly outwards.
- Place your fingertips on the floor.
- Exhale and bend your right leg, ensuring it tracks in line with your right foot, and straighten your left leg. Roll on to your left heel and point your toes up.
- Inhale and return to the centre.
- Exhale, bend your left leg and straighten your right leg. Roll on to your right heel and point your toes up.
- Inhale and return to the centre.
- Continue to flow from side to side. Inhale to the centre and exhale to the sides. Take care of your knees.

REPS: Four on each side.

CHANGE IT UP

If you want it more gentle...
For a less-strenuous version of this Move, see page 107.

MOVE 4: Advanced Lunge Flow

MOVE 5
ADVANCED HAMSTRING RELEASING

Hate stretching your hammies (but know you should)? This fast-moving sequence is the answer to keeping you entertained while preventing the dreaded 'pulled' hamstring that can mean months out of running, football or basketball. Usable both as a warm-up or cool-down sequence, it tests your flexibility, strength, balance and coordination. Just not your patience…

If you get twitchy sitting still and stretching your hamstrings then this active sequence may be the answer. The techniques will ask you to swing higher, fold deeper or drop lower than you did in the basic Hamstring Releasing Move, so how do you know that you are ready?

This Move demands above-average hamstring flexibility and a quick test will assess where you stand. 'Above average' is the ability to raise a straight(ish) leg to a 90-degree angle, or beyond, when lying on your back. Bend your left leg and place the foot on the floor, hold behind your thigh and ease it towards you. If you struggle here, stick with the basic Move until the hamstrings loosen up. Otherwise, feel free to explore the advanced versions.

Like many of the Advanced Moves, the techniques venture beyond the target muscle group to become whole-body movements, requiring a keen sense of balance, proprioception (the ability to sense the location of our limbs in space), coordination and core strength.

Swing and Tap and Pendulum challenge balance and proprioception while Inchworm adds a little upper body and core strength. Control the movement so you don't sink the hips in plank and bend the knees in the Downward Dog part if a ton of weight creeps into your shoulders. In fact, the knees can stay a little bent throughout the whole sequence; you will still get a great, effective hamstring stretch and it can feel much more comfortable than locking the leg straight.

TIP: MOVE TO THE 'EDGE' OF THE STRETCH AND OUT AGAIN, ESPECIALLY AT THE BEGINNING OF THE SEQUENCE.

STEP 1

SWING AND TAP

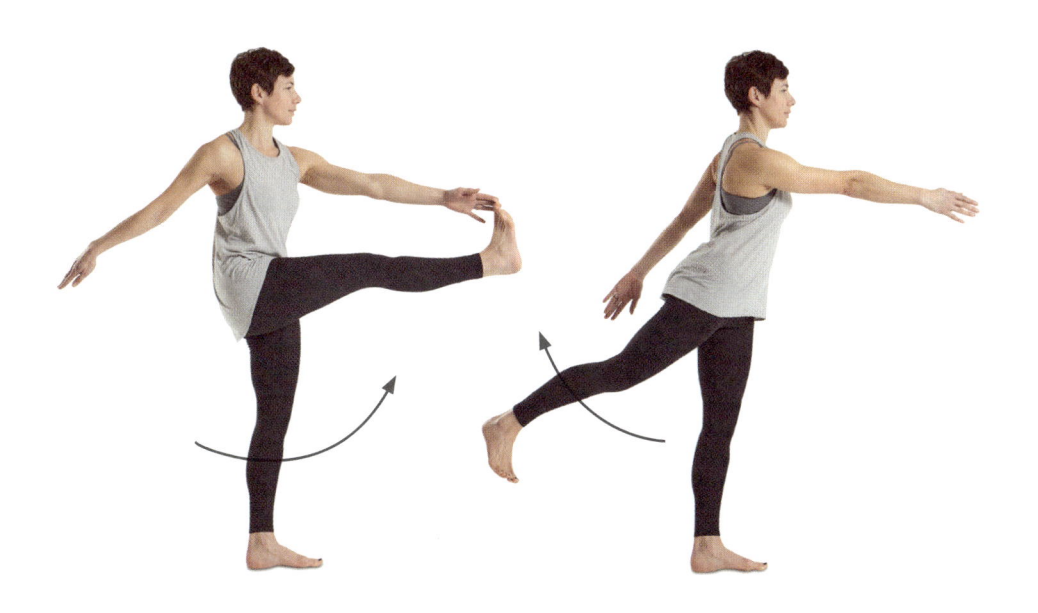

- Stand tall with your arms relaxed by your sides.
- Balance on your left leg and begin to swing your right leg forwards and backwards.
- Swing your arms in the opposite direction to your legs, as if walking or running.
- Now try to touch your right toes with your left hand on each swing.
- Breathe in and out as you swing.
- Complete your reps and switch legs, touching your left toes with your right hand.

REPS: Six–eight on each side.

PLAY: Try a few reps in slow motion to challenge balance and strength.

MOVE 5: Advanced Hamstring Releasing

STEP 2

PENDULUM

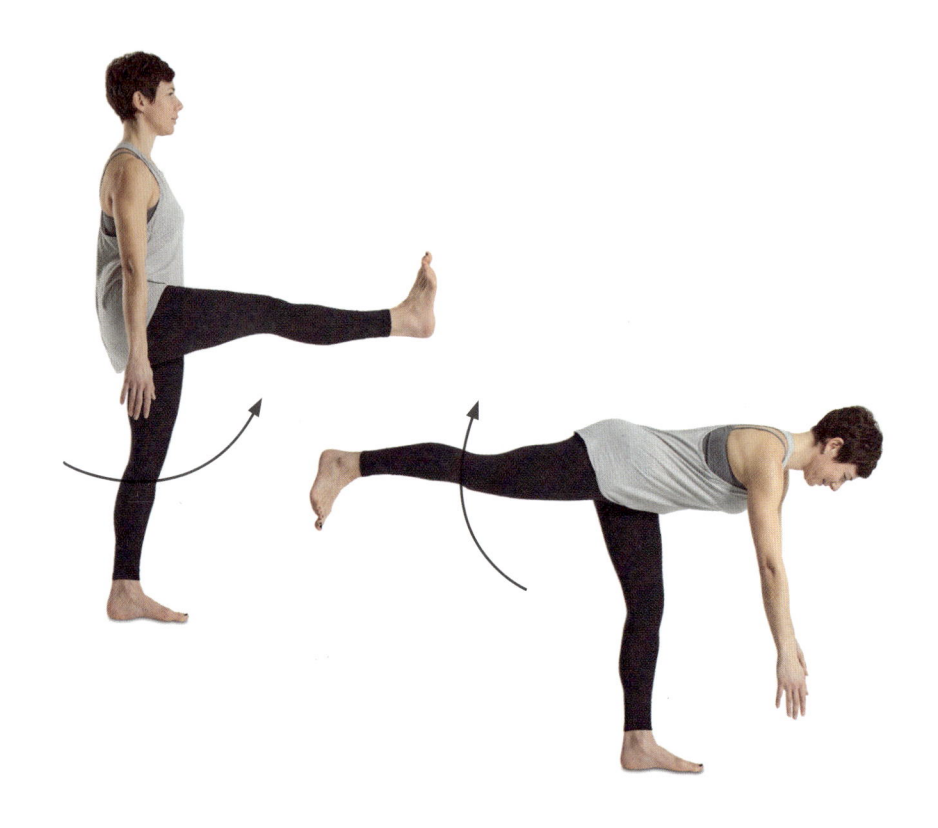

- Stand tall with your arms relaxed by your sides.
- Balance on your left leg, inhale and lift the right leg up to a 90-degree angle.
- Keeping your back straight, exhale, tip your body forwards and sweep the right leg back behind you. Let your arms dangle down.
- Continue to lift the right leg up and sweep it back, inhaling to lift and exhaling to sweep back.
- Complete the reps, then switch sides.

REPS: Four on each side.

STEP 3

TOE-UP WALKS

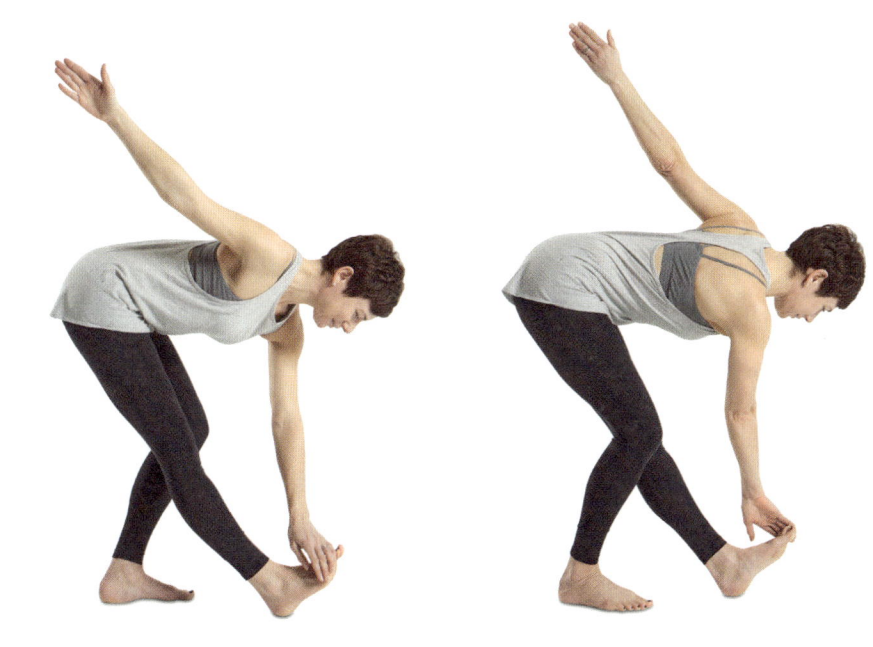

- Step your right foot forwards and point your toes up.
- Exhale and lean forwards over the right leg, keeping the back straight, then touch your toes with your left hand.
- Inhale and rise back up to standing.
- Step your left foot forwards and point your toes up.
- Exhale and lean forwards over the left leg, keeping the back straight, then touch your toes with your right hand.
- Continue to walk forwards, inhaling when upright and exhaling when leaning.

REPS: Four–six steps forwards.

MOVE 5: Advanced Hamstring Releasing

STEP 4

SWAYING DEEPER

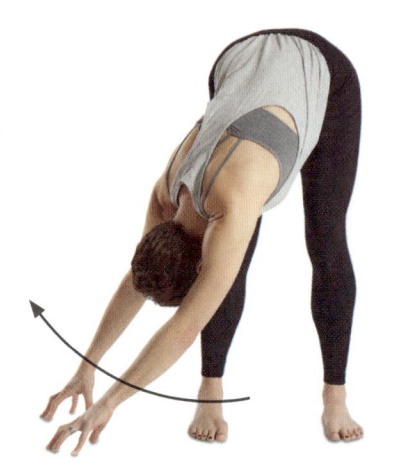

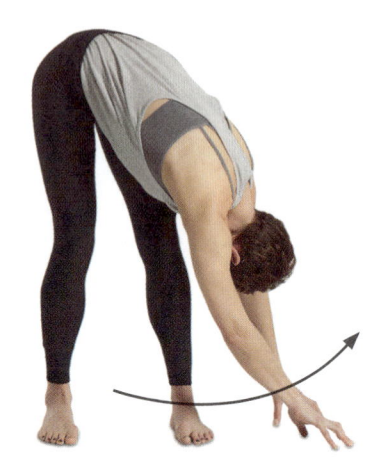

- Position your feet hip-width apart and relax your arms by your sides.
- Bend your knees slightly and roll down slowly towards the floor.
- Place your fingertips on the floor.
- Keeping your knees bent, sway your upper body slowly from side to side, walking your fingertips around to the right side and then the left.
- Breathe in and out as you sway.
- Exit by bending your knees deeper, pressing your hands on to your thighs, engaging the core and rising up with a straight back.

REPS: Sway for 10 seconds or longer.

PLAY: See how far round you can walk your fingertips.

STEP 5

INCHWORM

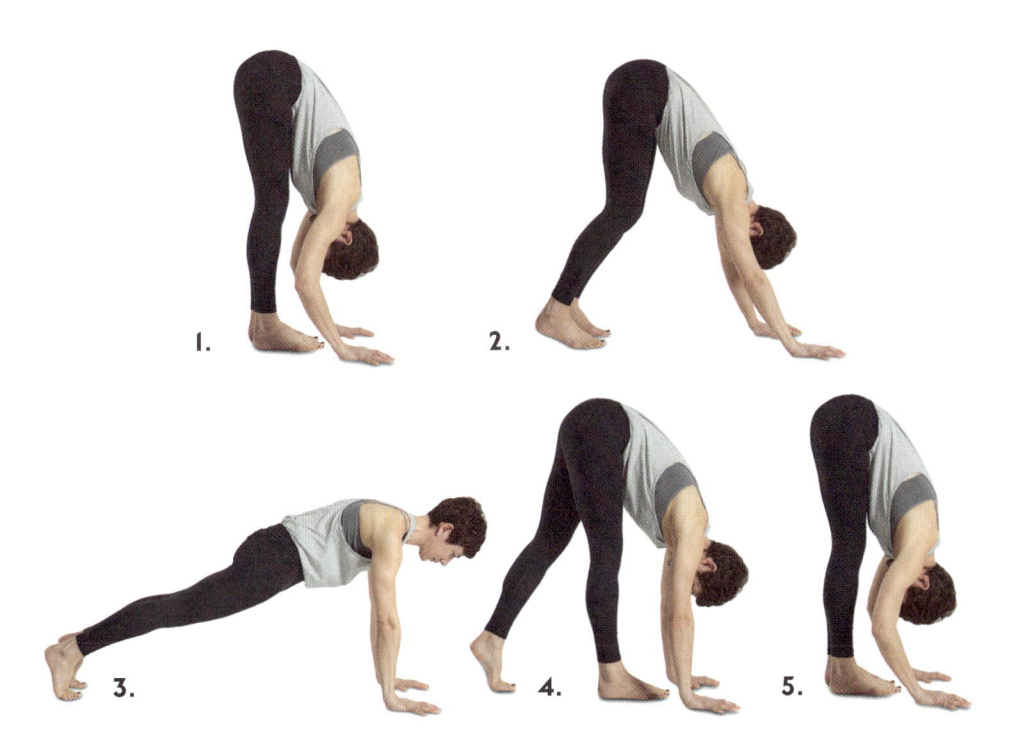

1.
2.
3.
4.
5.

- Stay folded forwards with your fingertips or hands on the floor.
- Keeping your legs straight, start walking your hands forwards until you straighten out into a plank and the back of your head is lined up with your hips and heels.
- Keeping your lefts straight start walking your feet up to your hands until you are back in a forward bend position.
- Complete the reps, continuing to move forwards.
- Breathe in and out as you transition through the movement.

REPS: Three.

PLAY: Walk your hands a little further past your shoulders in plank if the back and core are strong enough to support this.

MOVE 5: Advanced Hamstring Releasing

STEP 6

ADVANCED ROCK THE HAMMIES

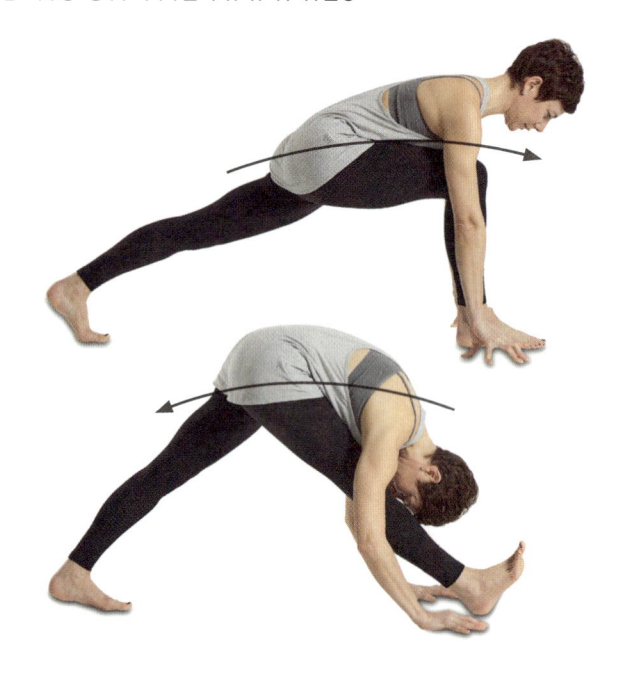

- Walk your hands back to your feet after the last Inchworm and take a big step backwards with your left leg to create a lunge.
- Place your fingertips on either side of your front foot and drop the hips into a lunge position.
- Inhale in the lunge. As you exhale, straighten your front leg and press your back heel down.
- Continue rocking back and forth by alternately bending and straightening your front leg.
- Complete the reps, then switch legs.

REPS: Four on each side.

CHANGE IT UP

If you want it more gentle...
For a less-strenuous version of this Move, see page 68.

MOVE 6
ADVANCED SHOULDER FLOSSING

When your mama told you to 'stop slouching' she was on to something. Shoulders are designed to move, not be stuck in a rounded position as we work, drive or mooch on the sofa. This sequence will keep them in tip-top condition for swimming, weightlifting or golf, and improve your posture by stretching the anterior shoulder muscles and 'pecs'.

Let's explore some deeper movements for the most mobile, manoeuvrable joints in the body: the wonderful shoulders.

Like the basic Shoulder Flossing Move you will need a strap, at least for half of the techniques. How long you keep the strap depends on your degree of shoulder flexibility. Hold on to it until Advanced Elbow Circles and then use this technique to experiment with how close you can walk your hands together. If you can't comfortably clasp your fingers, the strap can bridge this gap. This assessment is called 'Apley's scratch test' and is one method physical therapists use to test shoulder range of motion. Don't be surprised if it's (sometimes much) easier to grip on one side than the other. Just pause the flow on your tighter shoulder and hold for 30 seconds.

The grand plan of the Moves is to create more space in the body, so if you're struggling to grip and making the upper body lock up, go back to using the strap, at least until the shoulders loosen.

Move slowly and carefully in Up and Over – you always have the option to slide your hands wider apart on the strap. That extra space may make the movement smoother and more comfortable.

Keep an eye on your back in Bend and Flip, too. Weightlifters are familiar with straightening the back and engaging the core before standing upright as exiting with a flexed spine can load the lower back. Apply this thinking here and take a second to adjust the back.

Aside from simply shedding shoulder tension, this sequence will help prevent the rounded shoulders that lead to poor posture. It can also help provide that performance edge for sports that require superior shoulder flexibility, such as tennis, swimming or golf.

TIP: MOVE SLOWLY AND SMOOTHLY THROUGHOUT TO AVOID JARRING THE SHOULDERS.

STEP 1

UP AND OVER

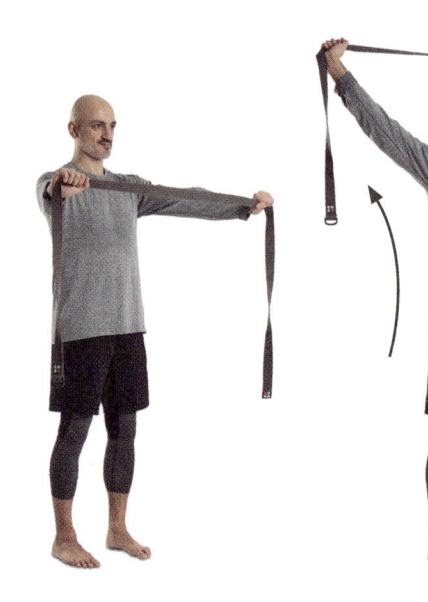

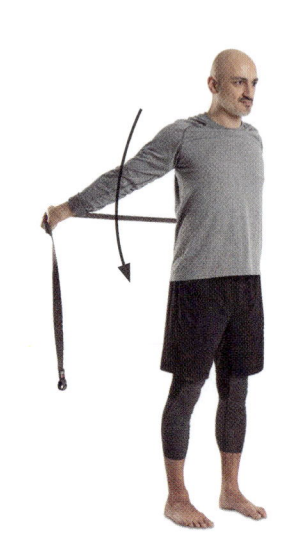

- Stand tall with your feet hip-width apart. Hold your strap in front of your body with your hands body-width, or wider, apart.
- Inhale, slowly raise the strap up and sweep it past your head, or as far as is comfortable.
- Exhale and sweep the strap back and down in front of your body.
- Continue, inhaling to raise the strap and exhaling to lower it.

REPS: Four.

PLAY: Want to improve your posture? Pause the movement as your strap moves just past your head, and take a few breaths.

STEP 2

BEND AND FLIP

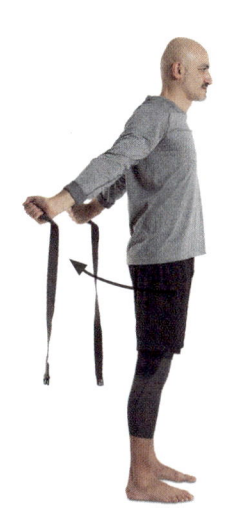

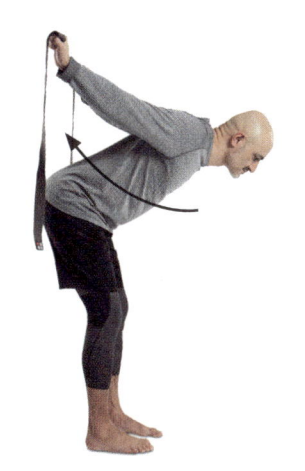

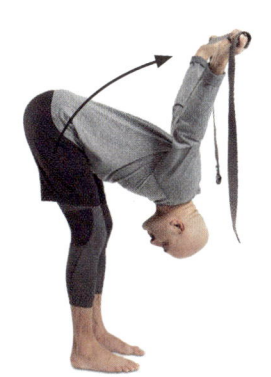

- Hold the strap behind your back.
- Change your grip so that your palms face your body.
- Keeping your back straight, exhale, bend your knees and tip forwards.
- Lift the strap and allow it to move forwards towards your head.
- To exit, bend your knees deeper, straighten your back, engage your core and, on an inhale, return to standing, allowing the strap to drop to the lower back.
- Continue, moving slowly and carefully. Inhale while returning to standing and exhale to fold forwards.

REPS: Four.

PLAY: If your strap flips right over your head and to the floor then you've flipped too far! Rise up and adjust your grip so that your hands are closer together.

MOVE 6: Advanced Shoulder Flossing

STEP 3

ADVANCED ELBOW CIRCLES

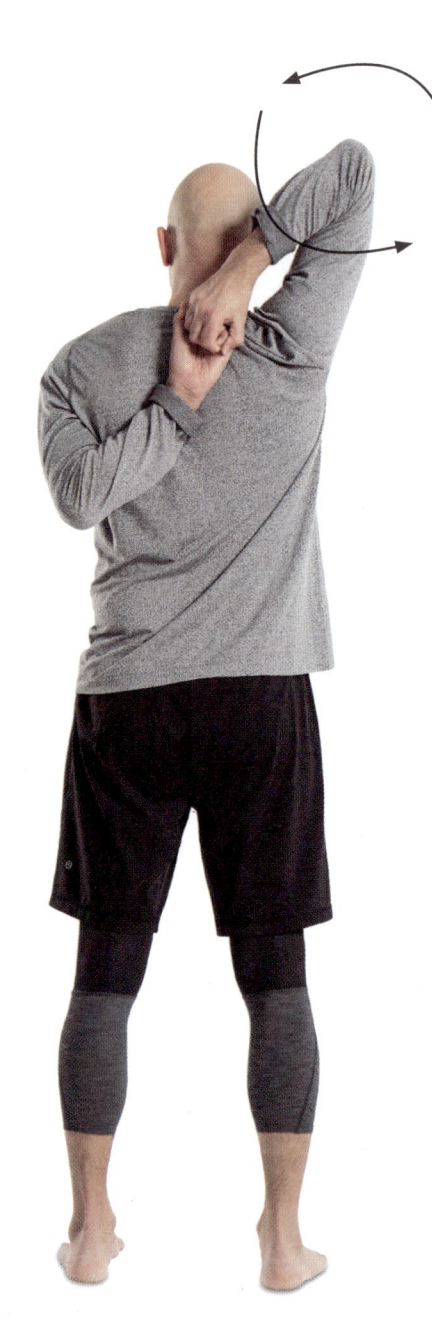

- You can drape a strap over your right shoulder, so it can be used if needed.

- Bend your right arm and drop your hand behind your back. Reach your left arm behind your lower back and wiggle it further up towards your should blades.

- Move your hands closer together. If the hands touch easily then clasp them. If not, use the strap to bridge the gap.

- Rotate the top elbow as if drawing small circles above your head.

- Breathe slowly in and out through the nose.

- Complete the reps, then switch arms.

REPS: 10 (five clockwise and five anticlockwise).

STEP 4

CLASPED SIDE STRETCH

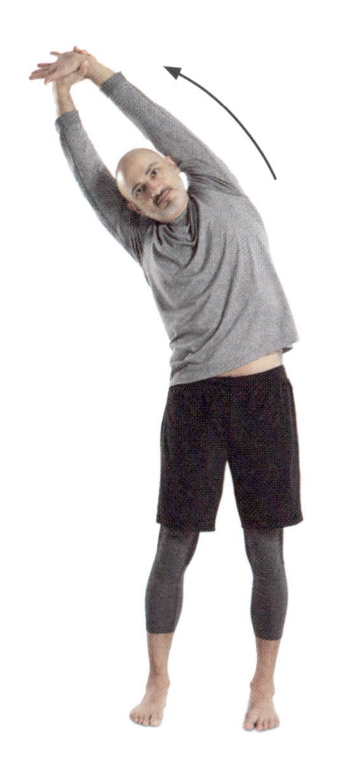

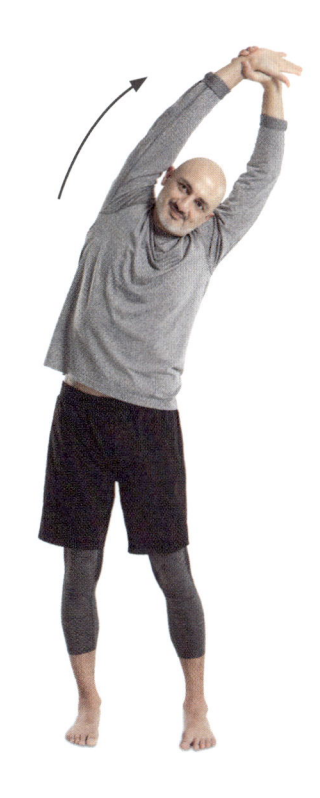

- Discard the strap and raise both arms above your head.
- Hold on to your left wrist with your right hand.
- Exhale, lean over to the right side and pull your left arm straighter.
- Inhale, return to the centre and release your hands.
- Hold on to your right wrist with your left hand.
- Exhale, lean to the left side and pull your right arm straighter.
- Inhale to the centre.
- Repeat to complete the reps.

REPS: Four on each side.

MOVE 6: Advanced Shoulder Flossing

STEP 5

WRAP AND SLIDE

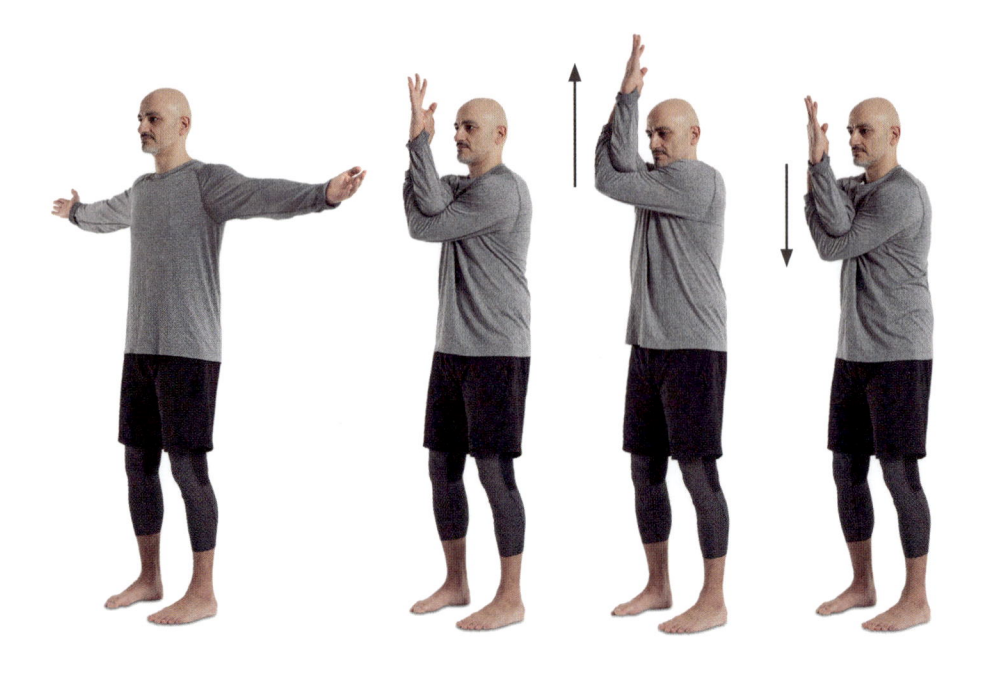

- Spread your arms wide.
- Cross your left arm over your right and bend both arms to bring the hands together.
- Slide both arms up, then slide then down inhaling to move up, exhaling to move down.
- Complete the reps. Unwrap, then wrap your right arm over your left and repeat the sliding movement on the other side.

REPS: Four on each side.

PLAY: Experiment with tucking your chin in and rounding or flexing your back a little while you slide.

STEP 6

WRAP AND ROTATE

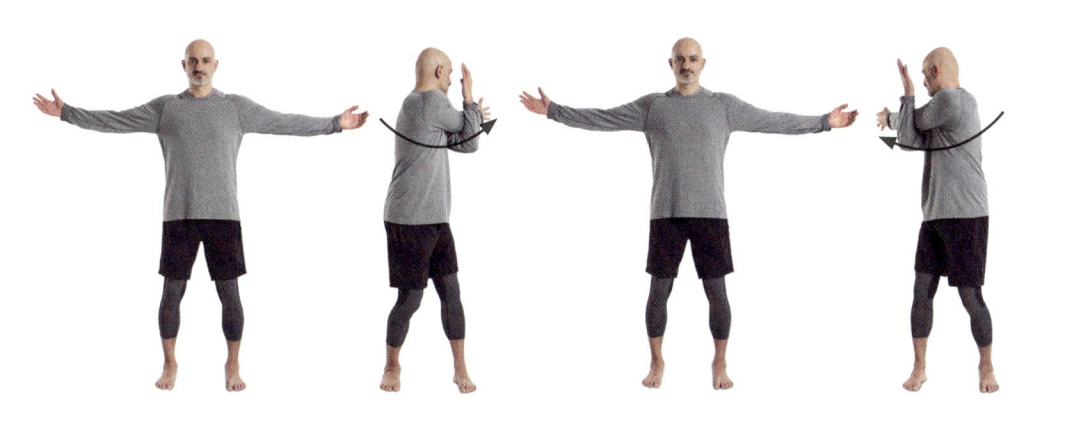

- Spread your arms wide.
- Sweep your right arm across your chest. Hug it close just above the elbow with the left hand, and on an exhale, rotate your upper body to the left.
- Inhale, return to the centre and spread your arms wide.
- Sweep your left arm across your chest. Hug it close with the right hand and on an exhale, rotate your upper body to the right.
- Complete the reps, moving slowly.

REPS: Four on each side.

CHANGE IT UP

If you want it more gentle...
For a less-strenuous version of this Move, see page 121.

MOVE 6: Advanced Shoulder Flossing

MOVING FORWARD

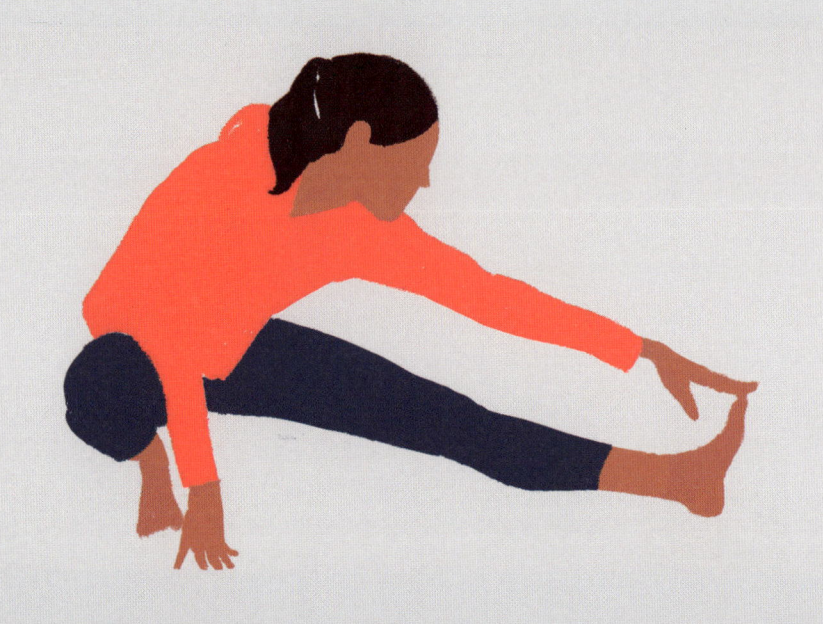

So, it's time to sign off. I really hope you enjoyed the journey to owning a body that feels good and moves well. Our purpose was not to enforce a strict exercise regime, but simply to remind ourselves of the pleasure of exploring movement; better flexibility was a happy by-product!

A lot of this exploratory movement we achieved through play. In a bid to reclaim some of that childhood mobility that our eight-year-old selves took for granted there were many playful flipping and squatting techniques mixed with yoga-inspired Cobras, Seals, Cats and Dogs. But behind all this play lies some serious heath benefits. Work, for many of us, is now cerebral, not physical, and this can mean hours sitting at a desk with precious little of the regular movement that the human body (and mind) needs to stay agile.

This means we need to factor in ways of moving in between and outside work to offset the sedentary time. Keeping the body moving is also highly beneficial to maintaining lower back health and for allowing you to immerse yourself in the sports you love without restriction or injury.

So now that you've come to the end of the book, where to next? The trick to maintaining your new-found mobility is 'little and often'. Don't set yourself the goal of working through all six Moves every day if, realistically, life won't let you.

Instead, do a bit here and there. Wake up and slide into Back Mobility by dropping the knees from side to side. Pre-empt running niggles by kicking off your jog with Hamstring Releasing. Keep a strap near the desk for Shoulder Flossing when the shoulders tighten up.

Those keen to continue beyond the Moves could take up a martial art; try a 'body balance', Pilates or yoga session or sample t'ai chi outside in the fresh air; the opportunities are everywhere.

Whatever happens going forward, good luck! Stay strong, be happy and keep moving.

OUR MOVERS

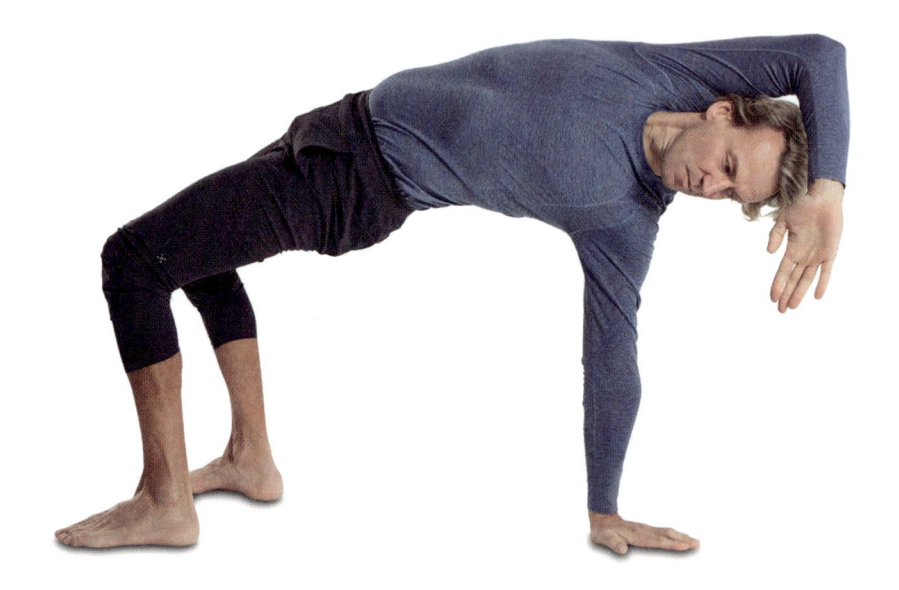

GEORGE SKUODAS

George teaches Animal Flow® – a system of building strength through motion by mimicking the movements of scorpions, crabs and other animals. He is also a personal trainer and yoga instructor. A former sailor, George began his sailing career at 17, turning professional in 1998. He represented Great Britain in the 1996 Atlanta Olympics and still competes internationally. George believes 'movement is part of everyday life' and is often found climbing trees, running with his dog, and flipping and gliding through Animal Flow® moves such as Reaches, Rolls and Kick Throughs.

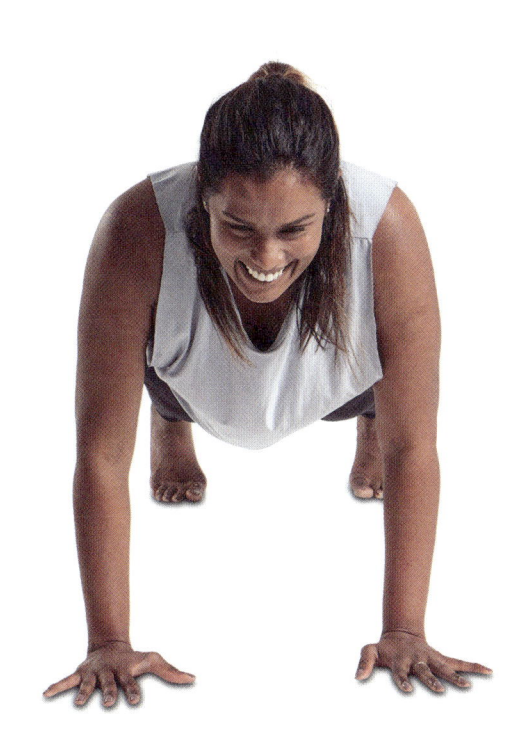

NISHA D'CRUZ

Global citizen Nisha was born in Singapore, worked in Perth and San Francisco, and now lives in Surrey, just outside London. Nisha teaches Spin®, Pilates and works as a fitness coach advising on both the physical and mental aspects of well-being. She also runs workshops and events with Surrey Total Health, a company comprising doctors, physiotherapists and nutritionists. Nisha is planning to combine a love of travel with fitness coaching by hosting her own mind and body health retreats in Europe.

OMAR BALUCH

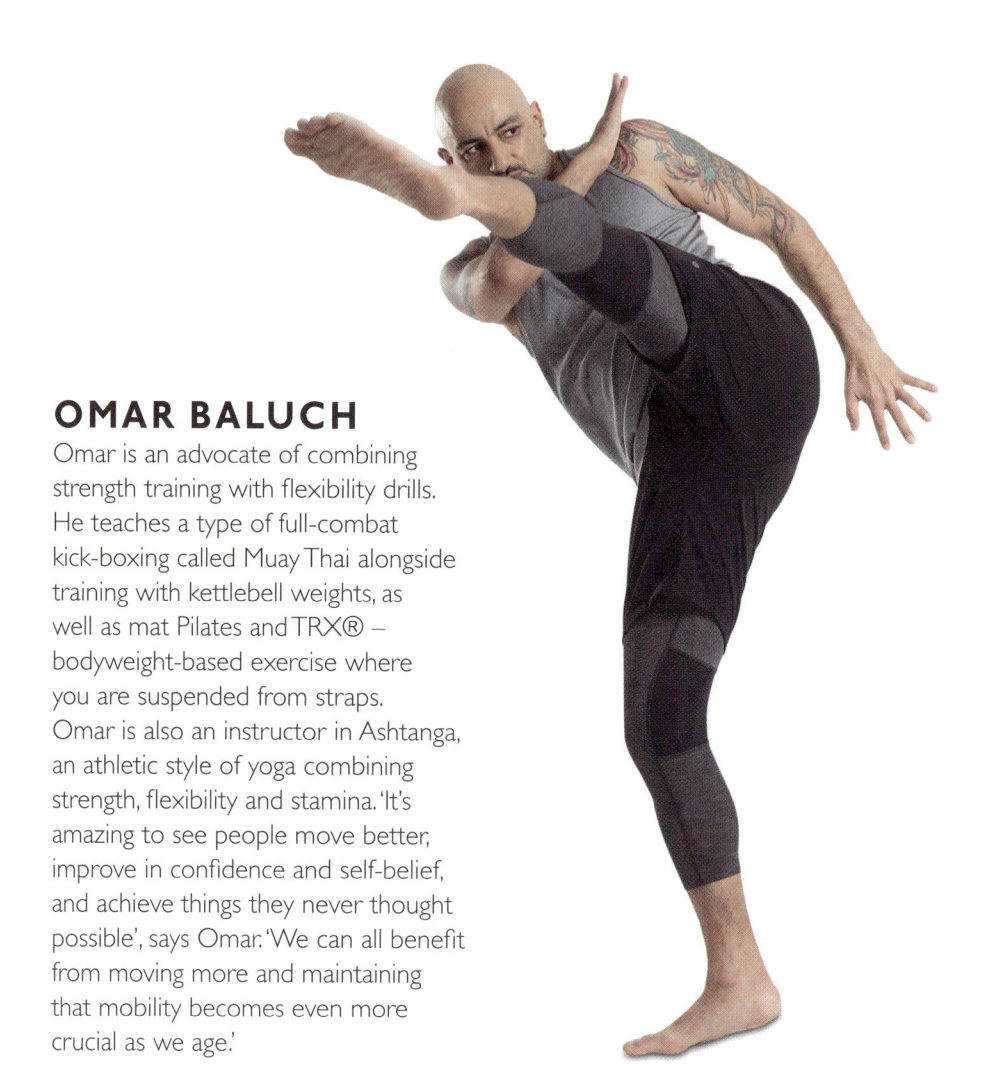

Omar is an advocate of combining strength training with flexibility drills. He teaches a type of full-combat kick-boxing called Muay Thai alongside training with kettlebell weights, as well as mat Pilates and TRX® – bodyweight-based exercise where you are suspended from straps. Omar is also an instructor in Ashtanga, an athletic style of yoga combining strength, flexibility and stamina. 'It's amazing to see people move better, improve in confidence and self-belief, and achieve things they never thought possible', says Omar. 'We can all benefit from moving more and maintaining that mobility becomes even more crucial as we age.'

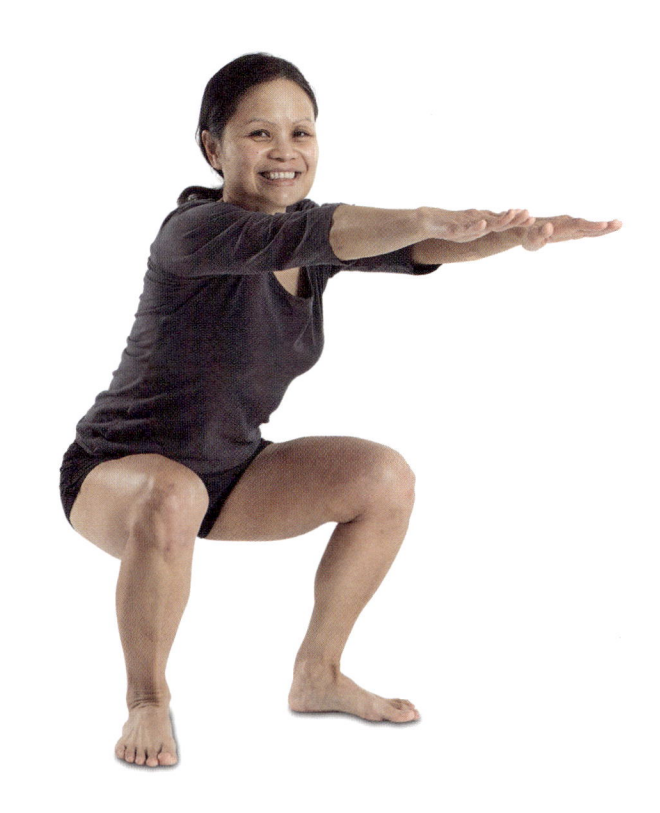

CINDY SIUKONEN

Californian-raised, London-based Cindy worked as a graphic designer for 17 years but recently turned freelance to launch Shortcrank, a business designing custom cycling and triathlon kit, blending her design savvy with a love of road cycling. Cindy originally converted to a healthy lifestyle of diet and exercise to lose weight but became hooked on the buzz of cycling, which she fits in around her freelance lifestyle (as long as the British weather obliges). 'Riding makes me feel good', explains Cindy. 'I get to explore, smell the air, feel the wind, meet new people, and most of all have coffee and cake!'

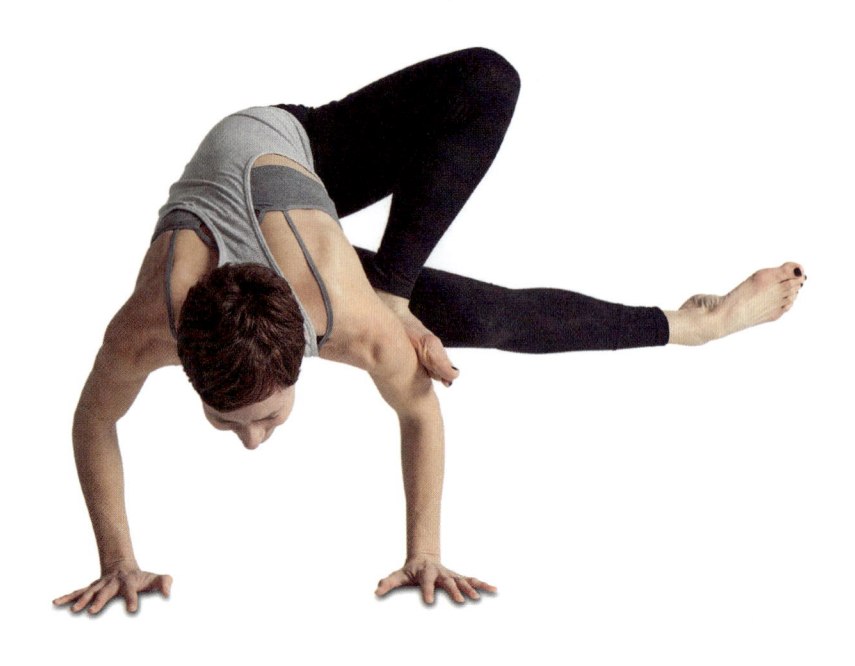

HANNAH JULIANO

Hannah's 'happy place' was once dancing to house music as a dedicated clubber. After a stint working in the fashion industry she found her way back to a different kind of movement in the form of yoga. Hannah signed up to a British Wheel of Yoga foundation course, later completing her 200-hour Yoga Alliance teacher training. She offers Seasonal Yoga, which changes its focus according to the seasons, and guided meditation sessions called Yoga Nidra ('Yoga Sleep'). 'If someone tells me that they feel less stressed, more relaxed or stronger than when they walked into the class,' says Hannah, 'then this makes me smile.'

ACKNOWLEDGEMENTS

I would like to thank my models Nisha D'Cruz, George Skuodas, Cindy Siukonen, Hannah Juliano and Omar Baluch who happily donated their time, energy and good vibes to this project. I was keen to find real people who truly believe 'Movement is Medicine' and work to promote the joy of movement, be it through Muay Thai kick boxing, yoga or encouraging others to find their inner ape, crab or crocodile in Animal Flow®. *Move* photographer Henry Hunt was ultra professional, and super chilled, which is an excellent combination when you have only hired the studio for a day, but have six separate shoots to complete with six different models. I'd also like to acknowledge Bloomsbury commissioning editor Matthew Lowing who encouraged me to break out of instructional manual mode and have fun writing *Move*. Finally, I'd like to thank my editor Sarah Skipper. We worked together on the ambitious 2017 title *The Stretching Bible* and Sarah is still hardworking, unflappable and a real sweetie, which is a much underrated quality.

AUTHOR BIO

Lexie Williamson is a fitness writer, yoga instructor and author of *The Stretching Bible, Yoga for Runners* and *Yoga for Cyclists*, all published by Bloomsbury. She also teaches anatomy and physiology to trainee yoga teachers.

British Wheel of Yoga (BWY) and Institute of Yoga Sports Science® trained, Lexie offers a practical, functional style of yoga mixing in Pilates and strength and conditioning, which is designed to appeal equally to men and women.

She specialises in tailoring yoga for sport, particularly running, cycling and triathlon, and works both with clubs and on a one-to-one basis with a range of endurance athletes, from newbie runners to Ironman™ veterans.

Lexie has also developed a range of techniques to help golfers improve their range of motion, and taught a range of other sportspeople, such as tennis players, rugby players and sprinters to become more supple, mobile and injury-resistant.

As a guest tutor on the BWY yoga teacher-training course, Lexie delivers sessions on anatomy and physiology and the science of flexibility, having studied exercise and sports science, and human anatomy and physiology.

A former magazine journalist and editor, Lexie has written for a wide range of publications, including *The Guardian, Women's Fitness, Cycling Weekly, Athletics Weekly* and *Runner's World*. She is a keen road cyclist and is a ride leader, and vice chairman, of Viceroys Triathlon Club in Surrey, UK. Lexie lives in Surrey with her husband Tom and three children Cameron, Finlay and Skye.

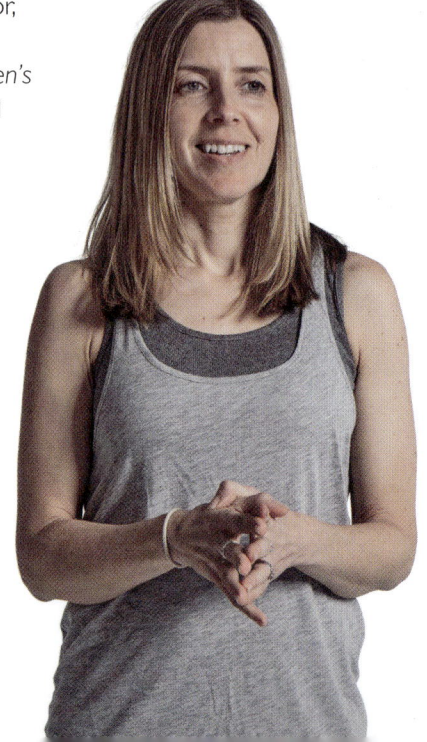